Prevention of Noncontact ACL Injuries

Edited by
Letha Y. Griffin, MD, PhD

Supported by the

 American Orthopaedic Society for Sports Medicine

 and the
National Athletic Trainers Association Research and Education Foundation

 and the
National Collegiate Athletic Association

 and the
Orthopaedic Research and Education Foundation

Workshop
Hunt Valley, Maryland
June 1999

 American Academy of Orthopaedic Surgeons
6300 North River Road
Rosemont, IL 60018

2000 – 2010

American Academy of Orthopaedic Surgeons

Prevention of Noncontact ACL Injuries

First Edition
Copyright © 2001 by the American Academy of Orthopaedic Surgeons

ISBN 0-89203-260-X
American Academy of Orthopaedic Surgeons

American Academy of Orthopaedic Surgeons

Contributors

Julie Agel, MA, ATC, Research Coordinator, Department of Orthopaedics, University of Minnesota, Minneapolis, Minnesota

Marjorie J. Albohm, MS, ATC, Director, Sports Medicine and Orthopaedic Research, Orthopaedics, Indianapolis, Indianapolis, Indiana

Elizabeth A. Arendt, MD, Associate Professor of Orthopedic Surgery, Department of Orthopedic Surgery, University of Minnesota, Minneapolis, Minnesota

Randall W. Dick, MS, FACSM, Senior Assistant Director of Health and Safety, National Collegiate Athletic Association (NCAA), Indianapolis, Indiana

William E. Garrett, Jr, MD, PhD, Frank C. Wilson Professor and Chairman, Department of Orthopaedic Surgery, University of North Carolina School of Medicine, Chapel Hill, North Carolina

James G. Garrick, MD, Director, Center for Sports Medicine, Saint Francis Memorial Hospital, San Francisco, California

Letha Y. Griffin, MD, PhD, Staff, Peachtree Orthopaedic Clinic, Team Physician, Georgia State University, Atlanta, Georgia

Timothy E. Hewett, PhD, Director of Applied Research, Adjunct Professor, Cincinnati Sportsmedicine Research and Education Foundation, Children's Hospital, University of Cincinnati, Cincinnati, Ohio

Laura J. Huston, MS, Senior Research Associate, Medsport, Section of Orthopaedic Surgery, University of Michigan, Ann Arbor, Michigan

Mary Lloyd Ireland, MD Orthopaedic Surgeon, Kentucky Sports Medicine, Lexington, Kentucky

Robert J. Johnson, MD, Professor of Orthopaedic Surgery, Department of Orthopaedics and Rehabilitation, University of Vermont, Burlington, Vermont

W. Benjamin Kibler, MD, Medical Director, Lexington Sports Medicine Center, Lexington Clinic, Lexington, Kentucky

Donald T. Kirkendall, PhD, Clinical Assistant Professor, Department of Orthopaedics, University of North Carolina, Chapel Hill, North Carolina

Scott Lephart, PhD, ATC, University of Pittsburgh, Pittsburgh, Pennsylvania

Contributors

Thomas N. Lindenfeld, MD,
Associate Director, Volunteer
Clinical Professor, University of
Cincinnati, Sportsmedicine and
Orthopaedic Center, Cincinnati,
Ohio

Bert R. Mandelbaum, MD,
Fellowship Director, Santa Monica
Orthopaedic and Sports Medicine
Group, Orthopaedic Surgery, Santa
Monica, California

Ralph K. Requa, MSPH,
Research Director, Center for
Sports Medicine, Saint Francis
Memorial Hospital, San Francisco,
California

Jennifer V. Riccobene, BA,
Research Assistant, Gait Analysis,
Cincinnati Sportsmedicine Research
and Education Foundation,
Cincinnati, Ohio

Bryan L. Riemann, MA, ATC,
University of Pittsburgh, Pittsburgh,
Pennsylvania

Carol C. Teitz, MD, Professor,
Orthopaedics and Sports Medicine,
University of Washington, Seattle,
Washington

Edward M. Wojtys, MD,
Professor, Department of
Orthopaedic Surgery, University of
Michigan, Ann Arbor, Michigan

Contents

Contents

Preface

The American Orthopaedic Society for Sports Medicine (AOSSM) is pleased to co-publish *Prevention of Noncontact ACL Injuries* with the American Academy of Orthopaedic Surgeons (AAOS). This publication provides physicians, other health professionals, coaches, and athletic administrators with information from recognized experts on the epidemiology, risk factors, prevention strategies, and other information related to noncontact anterior cruciate ligament (ACL) injuries.

AOSSM has long recognized the need for greater research and consensus on noncontact ACL issues. As an initial sponsor of the 1999 Hunt Valley Conference, AOSSM believed that a distinguished panel of experts could add to the scientific dialogue and provide clinical direction on this complex and controversial topic. Similarly, the Society's interest in sponsoring this publication is to help the broader sports medicine community more fully appreciate this significant problem and better safeguard athletes from sustaining ACL injuries.

While much research is still needed on ACL injury, this publication provides a foundation upon which we can build. We extend our appreciation to the participants in the Hunt Valley Conference and to the AAOS for making this publication a reality.

WALTON W. CURL, MD
AOSSM PRESIDENT

Foreword

Motivated by concern for the high incidence of anterior cruciate ligament (ACL) injuries occurring in 15- to 25-year-old athletes and realizing the significant physical, psychological, and financial implications of this injury, a group of orthopaedists, family practitioners, biomechanists, physical therapists, and athletic trainers met in Hunt Valley, Maryland, in June 1999 to examine the mechanisms of ACL injuries, risk factors predisposing athletes to injury, and existing ACL injury prevention programs. Funding for this meeting was obtained from the Orthopaedic Research and Education Foundation, and the American Orthopaedic Society for Sports Medicine; the National Athletic Trainers Association Research and Education Foundation; the National Collegiate Athletic Association; and the Sports Science Division.

The primary goal of the Hunt Valley meeting was to reach a consensus on prevention strategies for ACL injuries. Additional goals were to stimulate increased interest in injury prevention research and to foster educational efforts aimed at enhancing the public's awareness of this injury. Conference participants reviewed the existing literature on ACL risk factors and current prevention programs. This information served as background material for the discussion on risk factors for injury and the relationship of these factors to theoretical and existing prevention programs. Following this discussion, participants developed the consensus statements regarding prevention strategies for ACL injuries presented in this text.

After the Hunt Valley meeting, the Santa Monica ACL Prevention Group was formed. Using the principles agreed upon in Hunt Valley, this group created the "Prevent Injury and Enhance Performance (PEP) Program," an ACL injury prevention program that is sport-specific for soccer. The PEP program can be incorporated into the on-the-field, prepractice warm-up routine of the athlete. Sources for additional information on the PEP program and the other existing ACL prevention programs discussed in this text can be found in the Appendix.

LETHA Y. GRIFFIN, MD, PHD

Participants in the Hunt Valley Conference on ACL Prevention Strategies

Julie Agel, MA, ATC, Minneapolis, Minnesota
Elizabeth A. Arendt, MD, Minneapolis, Minnesota
Randall W. Dick, MS, FACSM, Indianapolis, Indiana
William E. Garrett, Jr, MD, PhD, Chapel Hill, North Carolina
James G. Garrick, MD, San Francisco, California
Letha Y. Griffin, MD, PhD, Atlanta, Georgia
Jo A. Hannafin, MD, PhD, New York, New York
Timothy E. Hewett, PhD, Cincinnati, Ohio
Laura J. Huston, MS, Ann Arbor, Michigan
Mary Lloyd Ireland, MD, Lexington, Kentucky
Robert J. Johnson, MD, Burlington, Vermont
W. Benjamin Kibler, MD, Lexington, Kentucky
Scott Lephart, PhD, ATC, Pittsburgh, Pennsylvania
Jack L. Lewis, PhD, Minneapolis, Minnesota
Thomas N. Lindenfeld, MD, Cincinnati, Ohio
Bert R. Mandelbaum, MD, Santa Monica, California
Patty Marchak, ATC, Dana Point, California
Aurelia Nattiv, MD, Los Angeles, California
Sandy Schultz, MS, ATC, Charlottesville, Virginia
Carol C. Teitz, MD, Seattle, Washington
Edward M. Wojtys, MD, Ann Arbor, Michigan

Santa Monica ACL Prevention Project Collaborators

Bert R. Mandelbaum, MD, Santa Monica, California
William E. Garrett, Jr, MD, PhD, Chapel Hill, North Carolina
Donald T. Kirkendall, PhD, Chapel Hill, North Carolina
Thomas P. Knapp, MD, Santa Monica, California
John Knarr, MS, PT, ATC, Los Angeles, California
Patty Marchak, ATC, Dana Point, California
Steve Sampson, MA, Los Angeles, California
Holly Silvers, MPT, Santa Monica, California
Steve Thomas, MPT, OCS, Santa Monica, California
Diane S. Watanabe, MA, ATC, Santa Monica, California

Acknowledgments

A note of appreciation to those who, recognizing the critical need for ACL prevention guidance for those participating in high-risk activities, gave of their time and expertise by attending the Hunt Valley Conference and to the sponsoring agencies for their financial and administrative support. Special recognition is given to Edward M. Wojtys, MD, who served as facilitator.

Chapter 1

Anterior Cruciate Ligament Injuries in Men and Women: How Common Are They?

James G. Garrick, MD
Ralph K. Requa, MSPH

Introduction

During the past 35 years, more than 3,500 indexed medical articles have been published covering the topic of anterior cruciate ligament (ACL) injuries. In spite of this plethora of information, surprisingly little is known regarding the basic epidemiology of this condition. Virtually every permutation of the diagnosis and treatment of this injury has been described, yet only rudimentary information exists regarding the frequency with which ACL injuries occur, the patterns with respect to age and sex, and the exact mechanism of injury.

Findings emerging from several studies indicate that female athletes are significantly more likely than male athletes to sustain ACL injuries in certain sports. This has stimulated a great deal of interest in both explaining this injury and preventing it—difficult tasks when the precise mechanism of injury has yet to be described (in either sex), and, except for the injuries documented in basketball, soccer, volleyball, team handball, and perhaps skiing, there are little or no data concerning injury rates in the general population or resulting from other activities.

This chapter reviews the evidence supporting a difference by sex in the incidence of ACL injuries, describes the activities in which such a difference exists, and identifies any temporal aspects of the occurrence of the injury in women.

Frequency of ACL Injury

Overall Incidence

In the general population, an ACL injury is a relatively uncommon occurrence. Data from the only study of incidence of ACL injuries in the general population suggest an annual incidence of approximately one injury for every 3,500 people, resulting in approximately 75,000 ACL injuries in the United States per year.[1] Others have estimated that 50,000 ACL reconstructions[2] are performed annually, compared with 120,000 total knee replacement procedures.[3]

Injury Distribution by Age

These figures may be misleading because ACL injuries are, for the most part, associated with sports activities in which the vast majority of participants are adolescents or young adults. In nearly every report, the largest segment of injuries is associated with sports. An example is a study by Daniel and associates,[1] wherein 70% of the injuries were the result of sports participation, with an average age at injury of 26 years. The authors also noted that only 5% of the ACL injuries occurred in patients either younger than 16 years or older than 45 years. Consistent with this is the fact that the average age of patients reported to have undergone ACL reconstructions is almost always in the 20s. Thus, nearly all ACL injuries appear to occur within a 30-year age bracket that encompasses roughly 47% of the population, resulting in a recalculated annual incidence of one injury for every 1,750 people in the age group at risk.

Further consider that in the general population study the "average ages" are calculated from the data sets that begin at about age 15 (few ACL injuries occur prior to this age) and may extend into the early 60s. Because of this highly skewed distribution, the vast majority of ACL injuries occur at ages younger than the average age for the series. This suggests that a segment of the population barely a decade in "width" (ie, between the ages of 15 and 25 years) is sustaining more than half of all the ACL injuries occurring in the United States—or one ACL injury annually for every 1,000 people in this age group.

Prevalence in Female Basketball and Soccer Players

Calculations based on rates presented in studies such as those of Arendt and Dick[4] and Zillmer and associates[5] project the annual number of ACL injuries in college soccer players at 237 (107 male, 130 female), college basketball players at 283 (62 male, 221 female), and high school basketball players at 5,773 (714 male, 5,059 female). These estimates are fairly consistent with the previously mentioned estimates of 75,000 total injuries, with 37,500 (one half) between the ages of 15 and 25 years, and 7,500 (20%) of those occurring in female athletes. Thus, soccer and basketball alone may be responsible for more than two thirds of the ACL injuries in women in this age group.

Sex as a Factor in Injury Rates

The Limits of Early Studies

Absent specific data from selected sports such as basketball, it would be easy to imagine that ACL injuries are overwhelmingly a male problem. Nearly all of the reports on diagnosis and treatment of these injuries contain a preponderance of male subjects. Starting with the original studies dealing with hemarthroses and ACL injuries and continuing with reports of various means of treatment, male participants have outnumbered female participants by at least two to one.

In 1980, in a study examining the initial presentation of ACL injuries, Noyes and associates[6] reported that only 13% of those with acute hemarthroses were women. Five years later, Daniel and associates[1] noted in a similar study that only 19% of the subjects were female. In one of the first articles on treatment, Marshall and associates[7] noted in 1982 that 29% of patients undergoing acute repairs were female. In the same year, Clancy and associates[8] also reported that women made up 29% of the group undergoing reconstruction, a proportion almost identical to the 31% reported by Shelbourne and associates[9] 8 years later. The presence of bilaterality of the ACL injury did not alter these ratios, with Harner and associates[10] reporting 29% female patients in the study group.

As was true with the original report by Daniel and associates, the majority of ACL injuries are associated with sports participation in virtually every report on diagnosis or treatment. Although the involvement of specific sports is almost always noted, most of the authors of these reports did not address the issue of differences by sex. Only when investigators looked at incidence by sport rather than total number of injuries did the suggestion of a disparity by sex emerge.

As early as 1980, Whitesides[11] noted that National Athletic Injury/Illness Reporting System (NAIRS) data dealing with college sports showed that among female basketball players, "sprains" were 50% higher and knee ligament injuries were 25% higher than in male basketball players. Zelisko and associates[12] reported an overall injury rate 1.6 times higher in female professional basketball players and knee injury rates that were more than two times higher. Chandy and Grana,[13] in a study of high school athletes, noted that girls' injury rates in basketball were 1.8 times those of boys; and, with roughly equal numbers of participants, female basketball players required knee surgery more than three times as often as boys. Zillmer and associates,[5] also studying high school basketball players, noted that the rate of major knee injuries among girls was 1.4 times that of boys.

Although these data, particularly the studies noting rates of surgical intervention, hint that ACL injuries may make up a substantial segment of knee ligament injuries, the issue of specificity of the structures injured is not addressed. With the earlier studies, this was probably a function of the fact that the diagnosis of ACL injuries lacked today's precision. The description of the Lachman test was not published until 1976, approximately the same time that diagnostic arthroscopy was becoming popular—both of which diagnostic tests led to our current level of recognition of the ACL problem.[14]

Emergence of the Significance of ACL Injury in Women

Reports suggesting a propensity for women to sustain ACL injuries surfaced in US sports medicine literature in 1985 with a report by Gray and associates,[15] which noted that ACL involvement among basketball injuries was 10 times higher in women than in men. In reporting the injuries occurring among basketball players competing in the Olympic tryouts, Ireland and Wall[16] noted that ACL injuries were more than four times more frequent in women than in men. Ferretti and associates[17] noted a similar preponderance of female volleyball players requiring ACL surgery.

Lindenfeld[18] was the first to examine this phenomenon in a prospective manner. In a study of youth soccer players, he noted that the knee ligament injury rate was three times higher in girls than in boys and that 80% of the ACL injuries involved girls even though girls represented only 43% of the total hours played. Arendt and Dick[4] studied National Collegiate Athletic Association (NCAA) injury reports and reported that ACL injury rates were 2.4 times higher in female soccer players and 4.1 times higher in female basketball players. In a study of Swedish soccer players, Roos and associates[19] also noted an increased ACL injury rate among female players, but the difference (1.4 times) was appreciably smaller than that reported in the United States. They also noted that the ACL injuries occurred at a younger age among the female players.

Although differences by sex in ACL injuries among recreational Alpine skiers have not been reported, competitive Alpine skiers display a disparity by sex (3.1-fold difference) comparable to that seen in the team sports described earlier.[20] Just as striking is the fact that 27% of the women with reconstructed ACLs reinjured the ACL graft—a rate more than twice that seen among the injured men (13%).

Different injury rates by sex have also been reported in team handball, a contact sport derived from soccer. In a study of team handball, Myklebust and associates[21] reported an injury rate in female players that was five times the rate in male players.

Unfortunately, there are few studies aimed at identifying specificity by sex across more than a single sport. A recent study[22] has attempted to close that gap in examining ACL injuries among midshipmen at the US Naval Academy. The authors examined not only the intercollegiate sports of basketball, soccer, and rugby, but also basketball and soccer at the intramural level as well as military training activities. They found a statistically significant difference between male and female injury rates ($P < 0.05$) in intercollegiate soccer, intramural soccer, and running the obstacle course. Higher, but not statistically significant, rates were also seen in female participants in intercollegiate basketball and rugby and in instructional wrestling in military training. Only intramural basketball failed to show a higher injury rate for women. Overall annual ACL injury rates among midshipmen showed a relative risk for women of 2.44.

Gymnastics, another sport associated with ACL injuries, does not lend itself to comparisons by sex because the events for men and women are dissimilar. An additional difficulty is the fact that among international competitors there is a substantial age difference between male and female athletes. College gymnastics (where ages are similar) has not as yet been the source of specific reports comparing male and female participants' ACL injury rates, although knee injury rates appear to be more than three times higher in women.[23]

Age and ACL Injury Risk in Women

Just as disquieting as the possible higher susceptibility of women to ACL injuries is the suggestion that the injuries in women are occurring at relatively younger ages than those sustained by men. The reason for this may lie in the fact that those activities associated with ACL injuries, especially in women, are team sports practiced almost exclusively at the high school and college levels, at least in the United States. Yet specific analyses of sports not exclusive to high schools and colleges have also produced suggestions that women with ACL injuries are younger than men with the same injuries, as documented by Roos and associates[19] among Swedish soccer players and suggested by Gerberich and associates[24] of US volleyball players.

Long-Term Significance of ACL Injuries

For some time it has been recognized that ACL injuries are not only immediately problematic because of functional instability but are also the source of long-term concerns. The association of posttraumatic degenerative joint disease with both ACL injuries and the often attendant meniscal injuries is well known. Equally accepted is the fact that such changes are likely to worsen with time. Thus, the earlier the injury occurs, the longer the time available to encounter these potentially disabling sequelae—an issue of some concern if women sustain these injuries at a younger age.

Conclusions

The single conclusion that appears inescapable from the previously mentioned studies is that in soccer, basketball, and probably team handball, female participants have statistically significant higher rates of ACL injuries than do male participants. In those studies where true rates have been calculated, the rate for women ranges from 2.4 times higher[4] to 9.5 times higher.[22]

Limitations of Available Data

Lack of True Epidemiologic Studies

The unfortunate lack of true epidemiologic studies—studies that calculate rates based on time-at-risk and that compare men's and women's participation in truly comparable activities—leads to drawing sweeping conclusions based on relatively small absolute numbers. Examining the aggregate total of women's ACL injuries in studies providing time-at-risk denominators[4,18,21,22] yields only 329 injuries (basketball 194, soccer 112, team handball 23), 87% of which arise from the NCAA study of Arendt and Dick.

Although the remainder of the reports contain few data allowing calculations of rates based on time-at-risk, there are no studies suggesting that men have a higher likelihood of ACL injuries (in the same sport) or that the ratios in other studies are unrealistically high. Still, in terms of absolute numbers, the higher rates of participation for men in activities associated with ACL injuries results in ACL-injured men outnumbering women by at least two to one.

Very Little Information on the Cause of Injury

Unfortunately, these studies and data provide little additional insight concerning the causes of ACL injuries. Soccer, basketball, and team handball are sports requiring quick stops and sudden turns, moves that are commonly cited as contributing to the mechanism of injury. These sports, especially basketball, also involve jumping, with a reasonably high likelihood of landing off balance because of the proximity of other players. Although the focus of fewer studies, volleyball[17] shares many activity characteristics with basketball and soccer and also appears to be a sport in which women are at higher risk for ACL injuries.

The injuries in Alpine skiing do not appear to occur at or near full extension but rather in positions of knee flexion—often greater than 90°. Whereas it is easy to envision the hamstrings being overwhelmed by the force of the quadriceps when the knee is in nearly full extension, as during a jump stop or cutting maneuver, it is more difficult to indict such a mechanism in a position where the mechanical advantage of the hamstrings is maximal and that of the quadriceps is appreciably compromised. Even though the quadriceps may be maximally contracted to combat uncontrolled knee flexion, one would expect significant hamstring activity to overcome hip flexion. These observations suggest that some additional, passive factor might be at least partially responsible for the higher rate of injuries in women, at least among skiers.

Prevention Studies

Efforts to examine the mechanism of injury have found their way into the literature only in the past few years. Likewise, it is only recently, and coinciding with the reports of higher injury rates among women, that studies dealing with prevention of ACL injury have been published. Of the 3,572 MedLine citations under the ACL topic heading, only 133 are subheaded "prevention," and fewer than 10 of those deal with prevention of the injury rather than prevention of some surgical complication.

The examination of factors potentially influencing the occurrence of ACL injuries is a step in the right direction. The search for effective injury prevention techniques will be furthered by increased knowledge of precise mechanisms of injury, biomechanical relationships, strength and flexibility issues, and hormonal influences. Such increased knowledge may lead to the prevention of ACL injuries in both men and women.

Fast Facts

Fact: In soccer, basketball, and volleyball, the rate of noncontact ACL injury is 2.4 to 9.5 times higher in women than in men.

Fact: Approximately 70% of ACL injuries in the United States are associated with sports participation.

Fact: The majority of ACL injuries occur between the ages of 16 and 45 years.

Fact: Women have a greater incidence than men of reinjury following knee reconstruction for ACL injuries.

Caution: One cannot generalize from the limited data in certain sports (basketball, soccer, and volleyball); therefore, the true incidence by sex of ACL injury remains unknown.

Begin: We must begin to collect data on the incidence of noncontact ACL injuries in a wide variety of sports, noting such factors as age, sex, and mechanism of injury.

Begin: Consider starting a registry for noncontact ACL injuries at the state and national level (high school, collegiate, and club) recording the age and sex of the injured athlete, as well as data on position played, field conditions, and other identifying data.

Begin: We must begin to collect better epidemiologic data at all levels of sports.

References

1. Daniel DM, Stone ML, Sachs R, Malcom L: Instrumented measurement of anterior knee laxity in patients with acute anterior cruciate ligament disruption. *Am J Sports Med* 1985;13:401-407.

2. Frank CB, Jackson DW: The science of reconstruction of the anterior cruciate ligament. *J Bone Joint Surg Am* 1997;79:1556-1576.

3. Poss R: Total joint replacement: Optimizing patient expectations. *J Am Acad Orthop Surg* 1993;1:18-23.

4. Arendt E, Dick R: Knee injury patterns among men and women in collegiate basketball and soccer: NCAA data and review of literature. *Am J Sports Med* 1995;23:694-701.

5. Zillmer DA, Powell JW, Albright JP: Gender-specific injury patterns in high school varsity basketball. *J Women's Health* 1992;1:69-76.

6. Noyes FR, Paulos L, Mooar LA, Signer B: Knee sprains and acute knee hemarthrosis: Misdiagnosis of anterior cruciate ligament tears. *Phys Ther* 1980;60:1596-1601.

7. Marshall JL, Warren RF, Wickiewicz TL: Primary surgical treatment of anterior cruciate ligament lesions. *Am J Sports Med* 1982;10:103-107.

8. Clancy WG Jr, Nelson DA, Reider B, Narechania RG: Anterior cruciate ligament reconstruction using one-third of the patellar ligament, augmented by extra-articular tendon transfers. *J Bone Joint Surg Am* 1982;64:352-359.

9. Shelbourne KD, Whitaker HJ, McCarroll JR, Rettig AC, Hirschman LD: Anterior cruciate ligament injury: Evaluation of intraarticular reconstruction of acute tears without repair: Two to seven year followup of 155 athletes. *Am J Sports Med* 1990;18:484-489.

10. Harner CD, Paulos, LE, Greenwald AE, Rosenberg TD, Cooley VC: Detailed analysis of patients with bilateral anterior cruciate ligament injuries. *Am J Sports Med* 1994;22:37-43.

11. Whitesides PA: Men's and women's injuries in comparable sports. *Phys Sportsmed* 1980;8(3):130-140.

12. Zelisko JA, Noble HB, Porter M: A comparison of men's and women's professional basketball injuries. *Am J Sports Med* 1982;10:297-299.

13. Chandy TA, Grana WA: Secondary school athletic injury in boys and girls: A three-year comparison. *Phys Sportsmed* 1985;13(3):106-111.

14. Torg JS, Conrad W, Kalen V: Clinical diagnosis of anterior cruciate ligament instability in the athlete. *Am J Sports Med* 1976;4:84-93.

15. Gray J, Taunton JE, McKenzie DC, Clement DB, McConkey JP, Davidson RG: A survey of injuries to the anterior cruciate ligament of the knee in female basketball players. *Int J Sports Med* 1985;6:314-316.

16. Ireland ML, Wall C: Abstract: Epidemiology and comparison of knee injuries in elite male and female United States basketball athletes. *Med Sci Sports Exerc* 1990;22(Suppl):S82.

17. Ferretti A, Papandrea P, Conteduca F, Mariani PP: Knee ligament injuries in volleyball players. *Am J Sports Med* 1992;20:203-207.

18. Lindenfeld TN, Schmitt DJ, Hendy MP, Mangine RE, Noyes FR: Incidence of injury in indoor soccer. *Am J Sports Med* 1994;22:364-371.

19. Roos H, Ornell M, Gardsell P, Lohmander LS, Lindstrand A: Soccer after anterior cruciate ligament injury: An incompatible combination? A national survey of incidence and risk factors and a 7-year follow-up of 310 players. *Acta Orthop Scand* 1995;66:107-112.

20. Stevenson H, Webster J, Johnson R, Beynnon B: Gender differences in knee injury epidemiology among competitive alpine ski racers. *Iowa Orthop J* 1998;18:64-66.

21. Myklebust G, Maehlum S, Holm I, Bahr R: A prospective cohort study of anterior cruciate ligament injuries in elite Norwegian team handball. *Scand J Med Sci Sports* 1998;8:149-153.

22. Gwinn DE, Wilckens JH, McDevitt ER, Ross G, Kao TC: Abstract: Relative gender incidence of anterior cruciate ligament injury at a military service academy. *66th Annual Meeting Proceedings*. Rosemont, IL, American Academy of Orthopaedic Surgeons, 1999, p 117.

23. Hutchinson MR, Ireland ML: Knee injuries in female athletes. *Final Program Book of Abstracts and Outlines, 21st Annual Meeting*. Rosemont, IL, American Orthopaedic Society for Sports Medicine, 1995.

24. Gerberich SG, Luhmann S, Finke C, Priest JD, Beard BJ: Analysis of severe injuries associated with volleyball activities. *Phys Sportsmed* 1987;15(8):75-79.

Chapter 2
Shoe/Surface Considerations

Randall W. Dick, MS, FACSM

The Surface

For more than 30 years, researchers have been assessing the influence of the playing surface on injury rates. Studies regarding the contribution of the playing surface to injury rates in football as well as in soccer and tennis are reviewed here.

Football

With the advent of artificial grass surfaces and the growth in popularity of football, studies evaluating injuries on artificial and natural grass football surfaces were frequent in the 1980s. Findings varied significantly by study. While Stevenson and Anderson[1] found a higher relative risk (1.8) of injury on artificial turf in a randomized study of collegiate intramural teams, and Powell and Schooman[2] found a significantly higher risk of knee sprains on AstroTurf in a 10-year review of National Football League game injuries, Nicholas and associates[3] found no significant differences between grass- and artificial turf-related injuries in a 20-year analysis of one National Football League team. Two review articles at the end of the decade provided a summary of these studies: Nigg and Segesser[4] noted that in football, artificial surfaces produced nonsevere injuries (eg, abrasions) more frequently than did natural grass. Severe injuries, however, seemed to occur as frequently on natural grass as on artificial turf. Skovron and associates[5] noted that football play and practice on artificial surfaces was probably responsible for an increase in the relative risk of injury to the lower extremity.

However, football may not be the best sport in which to evaluate the effect of the playing surface on injuries. As Ekstrand and Nigg[6] pointed out, severe injuries in football typically occur in collision situations that are often independent of the surface.

Soccer and Tennis

The effect of shoe/surface interaction on injury rates in soccer and tennis has also been examined. Studies have identified the playing surface as contributing to injury in both sports, with the differences in injury frequency suggested to be directly related to differences in the frictional properties of the surfaces.[4,6]

The Shoe/Surface Interaction

These studies focused on the playing surface as the contributor to injury, despite the fact that the friction associated with a foot-plant injury involves two surfaces. The concept of a "release coefficient," a quantitatively measured force-to-weight ratio of shoe/surface interaction developed by Torg and associates[7] in the early 1970s, was often ignored.

More recently, the contribution of the shoe to the shoe/surface interaction has been investigated. Heidt and associates[8] evaluated the shoe/surface interaction of 15 athletic shoes and a variety of surface conditions in a laboratory setting. Using a release coefficient (force-to-weight ratio) established by Torg and associates,[7] 33 (73%) of the shoe/surface combinations in this study were rated "unsafe" or "probably unsafe." Shoes tested in conditions for which they were not designed exhibited reproducible excessive or extreme minimal friction characteristics that may have safety implications.

Relationship of Shoe/Surface Interaction to ACL Injury

Scandinavian researchers assessing injuries in the hard-floor sport of team handball have reported that a major risk factor for noncontact anterior cruciate ligament (ACL) injury is the high friction between shoes and playing surfaces. Strand and associates[9] found retrospectively that 66% of 144 reported ACL injuries in Norwegian team handball players were noncontact injuries. A majority of ACL injuries to female athletes occurred on synthetic surfaces, and the risk of ACL injury when playing on parquet (wood) was considerably lower. The authors concluded that a major risk factor was high friction between shoes and playing surfaces. Myklebust and associates[10] found that 95% of 93 cruciate injuries (primarily ACLs) in Norwegian handball players involved no contact between players and that activities involving significant friction between shoe and floor caused 55% of the injuries.

A prospective 3-year study of more than 3,000 high school football players[11] showed that the cleat design producing the highest torsional resistance in the laboratory was associated with a significantly higher rate of ACL injury.

The complex nature of shoe/surface interactions (and perhaps other contributing factors, such as braces and foot orthotics) makes them difficult to quantify, but the concept of a release coefficient is a good start. Friction, which involves the interaction of two distinct surfaces, appears to be an important consideration in assessing surface-related injury risk.[12] Therefore, both components of the shoe/surface system must be considered when making modifications to the system in an attempt to reduce injury rates.

The Balance Between Performance and Safety

Another complicating factor to consider is the balance between performance and safety. Characteristics of shoes and surfaces can affect an athlete's performance. Ekstrand and Nigg[6] noted that frictional resistance must be held within an optimal range that both minimizes rotational friction for the purpose of decreasing injury incidence and keeps translational friction high enough for optimal athletic performance. Higher levels of fixation are generally associated with better performance but also with a higher injury risk. Therefore, although the shoe/surface interaction as a risk factor for ACL injury is modifiable, the solution that results in a safer environment may exclude that which offers optimal performance.

Fast Facts

Fact: The interaction of the athlete's shoe with the playing surface influences performance and knee injury rates. Greater friction between shoes and surface provides better traction for sport performance but increases the risk of knee ligament injury.

Caution: Remember that weather often affects outdoor playing surfaces.

Begin: Develop the "ideal shoe" for different surfaces or the "ideal surface" for any shoe, ie, one that decreases knee ligament injuries but maintains performance advantages.

References

1. Stevenson M, Anderson B: The effects of playing surfaces on injuries in college intramural touch football. *J Natl Intramural Recreation Sports Assoc* 1981;5:59-64.

2. Powell JW, Schootman M: A multivariate risk analysis of selected playing surfaces in the National Football League: 1980 to 1989. An epidemiologic study of knee injuries. *Am J Sports Med* 1992;20:686-694.

3. Nicholas JA, Rosenthal PP, Gleim GW: A historical perspective of injuries in professional football. Twenty-six years of game-related events. *JAMA* 1988;260:939-944.

4. Nigg BM, Segesser B: The influence of playing surfaces on the load on the locomotor system and on football and tennis injuries. *Sports Med* 1988;5:375-385.

5. Skovron ML, Levy IM, Agel J: Living with artificial grass: A knowledge update. Part 2: Epidemiology. *Am J Sports Med* 1990;18:510-513.

6. Ekstrand J, Nigg BM: Surface-related injuries in soccer. *Sports Med* 1989;8:56-62.

7. Torg JS, Quedenfeld TC, Landau S: The shoe-surface interface and its relationship to football knee injuries. *J Sports Med* 1974;2:261-269.

8. Heidt RS Jr, Dormer SG, Cawley PW, Scranton PE Jr, Losse G, Howard M: Differences in friction and torsional resistance in athletic shoe-turf surface interfaces. *Am J Sports Med* 1996;24:834-842.

9. Strand T, Tvedte R, Engebretsen L, Tegnander A: Anterior cruciate ligament injuries in handball playing: Mechanisms and incidence of injuries [in Norwegian]. *Tidsskr Nor Laegeforen* 1990;110:2222-2225.

10. Myklebust G, Maehlum S, Engebretsen L, Strand T, Solheim E: Registration of cruciate ligament injuries in Norwegian top level team handball: A prospective study covering two seasons. *Scand J Med Sci Sports* 1997; 7:289-292.

11. Lambson RB, Barnhill BS, Higgins RW: Football cleat design and its effect on anterior cruciate ligament injuries: A three-year prospective study. *Am J Sports Med* 1996;24:155-159.

12. Levy IM, Skovron ML, Agel J: Living with artificial grass: A knowledge update. Part 1: Basic science. *Am J Sports Med* 1990;18:406-412.

Chapter 3

The Effect of Prophylactic Knee Bracing on Injury Prevention

Marjorie J. Albohm, MS, ATC

Introduction

Knee brace functionality and related issues of efficacy have long been an area of controversy in sports medicine. Motivated by concerns about false claims by manufacturers, research addressing these issues has increased significantly in recent years. As a result, much more is known about knee braces, resulting in scientific documentation of brace function and leading to design improvements and revised recommendations for use based on results of controlled clinical trials. Although this research emphasis has expanded the scientific body of knowledge on this subject, many questions remain unanswered. For example, the effect of knee bracing on proprioception is not fully understood, nor has knee bracing in women been adequately studied.

Types of Bracing

Knee bracing in the athlete occurs in two basic forms: prophylactic bracing and functional bracing. The prophylactic knee brace is designed primarily to absorb direct or indirect stress encountered during an athletic maneuver to prevent or reduce the severity of knee injuries. The functional brace was originally designed to enhance knee stability in patients with an anterior cruciate ligament (ACL)-deficient knee.

Prophylactic Knee Braces

In 1979, Anderson and associates[1] reported on a knee brace, called the "Anderson knee stabler," designed to protect knees from collateral ligament injury. This brace and ones that followed were termed "prophylactic" knee braces. There are two basic design types of prophylactic knee braces. The first consists of a lateral bar design with a single axis, dual axis, or polycentric hinges fitted with a hyperextension stop. The second type consists of plastic cuffs with polycentric hinges. This type is often custom fitted. Results of research on the effectiveness of these braces are varied.

Clinical Brace Research Teitz and associates[2] collected data from National Collegiate Athletic Association (NCAA) Division I schools, 71 in 1984 and 61 in 1985, to determine if the use of preventive braces for the knee was associated with a decrease in either the severity or incidence (or both) of knee injuries in collegiate football players.

Data received via survey questionnaires from 6,307 players in the 1984 portion of the study and from 5,445 players in the 1985 study were grouped according to position played. Players with a prior knee injury were excluded. The braces used had a common hinged stay.

Results of this survey study indicated that players who wore knee braces had significantly more injuries to the knee than players who did not (in 1984, 11.0% compared with 6.0%; in 1985, 9.4% compared with 6.4%) ($P < 0.001$). The injuries reported included those to the medial collateral ligament, the ACL, and the meniscus, incurred separately or in combination.

A study published by Hewson and associates[3] in 1986 evaluated the effectiveness of the Anderson knee stabler in reducing the number and severity of knee injuries in football players at the University of Arizona. Data were collected over a 4-year period (1981-1984) on all offensive and defensive linemen, linebackers, and tight ends. Total injury exposure, counted as one exposure for each player at each practice session or game, equaled 28,191 for the brace group and 29,293 for the control group. The data analyzed were days lost from practice or games, the player's position, the type and severity of injury, and the rate of injury per 100 players per season. Of the players at risk, the type and severity of injury in nonbraced and braced groups were similar.

In 1987, Rovere and associates[4] reported results of a study evaluating knee injury rates in a major college football team during 2 years when all players were required to wear laterally placed prophylactic knee braces during all practices and games. The results indicated that the incidence of knee injuries was higher when braces were worn compared to a similar period when braces were not worn. There was also an increased number of ACL injuries during the time when braces were worn. The study concluded that the efficacy of prophylactic knee braces in preventing knee injuries in collegiate football was highly questionable.

A study by Grace and associates,[5] published in 1988, evaluated 588 high school football players over two seasons to determine the effectiveness of prophylactic knee bracing on lower extremity injury. Two hundred forty-seven athletes who wore single-hinged braces and 83 who wore double-hinged braces were paired for the same season of play with 250 athletes who did not wear braces. The 53 injuries of the knee that occurred were significantly more frequent ($P < 0.001$) in the group that wore single-hinged braces than in the matched, nonbraced group. There was also a dramatic increase ($P < 0.001$) in the number of injuries to the ankle and foot in athletes who wore braces. Results of this study question the efficacy of the braces that were studied and call attention to the potentially adverse effect of the braces on adjacent joints.

Sitler and associates[6] reported in 1990 the results of a prospective randomized study to determine the efficacy of prophylactic knee bracing in reducing the frequency and severity of acute knee injuries in football. The participants in the study were 1,396 cadets at the United States Military Academy, who experienced a total of 21,570 athlete exposures in the 1986 and 1987 fall intramural tackle football seasons. Results of the study indicated that the use of prophylactic knee braces significantly reduced the frequency of knee injuries, both in the total number of subjects injured and in the total number of medial collateral ligament injuries incurred. However, the reduction in the frequency of knee injuries was dependent on player position. Defensive players who wore prophylactic knee braces had statistically fewer knee injuries than players who served as controls. The severity of medial collateral ligament and ACL injuries was not significantly reduced with the use of prophylactic knee braces.

Albright and associates[7] in a survey study evaluated the effectiveness of preventive braces on medial collateral ligament sprains in NCAA Division I college football players. Position, strength, type of session, and daily brace wear were recorded. Nine hundred eighty-seven Big Ten players generated 155,772 knee exposures over the course of the study; 50% of those players wore braces. Although noticeable differences existed in injury rates for the braced and nonbraced knees during practice sessions, when the factors of position, strength, and session were considered, a statistically significant lower injury rate was not demonstrated. For starters and substitutes in the line positions, as well as the linebackers and tight ends, there was a consistent trend toward lower injury rates in both practices and games. The braced players in the skill positions (backs, kickers), at least during games, exhibited a higher injury rate.

A review of six studies utilizing epidemiologic criteria to evaluate the effect of prophylactic knee bracing in football, conducted by Garrick and Requa,[8] concluded that there is very little agreement about the effects of prophylactic knee bracing in football. Many of the studies demonstrated methodologic faults with uncontrolled variables, bias in selecting cases and controls, and variations in defining injury and exposure. The reviewers could find no statistical consensus among the studies.

Laboratory Studies Because of the formidable methodologic and logistic barriers to conducting well-controlled prospective bracing studies of sufficient population size to establish or refute brace efficacy, it is necessary to consider the laboratory evaluation of prophylactic knee bracing. Most of the early laboratory work involved cadavers. Mechanical surrogate leg models were introduced to overcome cadaver shortcomings. Brown and associates[9] and France and Paulos[10] concluded, however, that there is no ideal way to truly evaluate bracing in the laboratory because of the inability to simulate on-field situations. Large numbers are also needed epidemiologically to provide meaningful data.[11]

Functional Knee Braces

Controversy exists regarding the effectiveness of functional knee braces. Research has addressed a static and functional assessment of these devices. Subjectively, patients report that braces are effective in reducing, but not eliminating, subluxation events. However, controlled studies have not verified these personal accounts.[12]

Ryder and associates[13] reported that functional knee braces appear to have a beneficial strain-shielding effect on the ACL for anteriorly directed loads and internal-external torques applied to the tibia. This effect, however, appears to decrease as the magnitude of these anteriorly directed loads and torques increases.[13] Functional braces have also been reported to modify electromyographic activity and timing in skiers who have ACL injuries.[14] The prophylactic significance of these early data has not yet been established.

Functional braces do appear to be effective in controlling motion in the ACL-deficient knee at low loads. During predicted maneuvers in controlled situations, these braces appear to be effective. In situations in which high loads are encountered or when the load is applied in an unpredictable fashion, the braces appear to fail.[13]

Conclusion

Additional controlled clinical trials are needed to determine the efficacy of prophylactic and functional knee bracing. The multiple variables associated with conducting these studies create significant challenges for investigators. Multicenter studies enrolling large numbers of athletes are needed.

Fast Facts

Fact: Prospective, controlled, randomized studies evaluating the effectiveness of knee braces in preventing noncontact ACL injuries are limited.

Fact: No conclusive studies demonstrate the effectiveness of functional knee braces in preventing noncontact ACL injuries.

Fact: It is difficult to evaluate the psychologic value of a knee brace.

Caution: Use caution when prescribing prophylactic braces for noncontact ACL injuries. Do not tell the athlete that the brace has been definitely shown to protect against injury.

Begin: Additional studies are needed on the proprioceptive and psychologic value of knee braces.

References

1. Anderson G, Zeman SC, Rosenfeld RT: The Anderson knee stabler. *Phys-Sportsmed* 1979;7(6):125-127.

2. Teitz CC, Hermanson BK, Kronmal RA, Diehr PH: Evaluation of the use of braces to prevent injury to the knee in collegiate football players. *J Bone Joint Surg Am* 1987;69:2-9.

3. Hewson GF Jr, Mendini RA, Wang JB: Prophylactic knee bracing in college football. *Am J Sports Med* 1986;14:262-266.

4. Rovere GD, Haupt HA, Yates CS: Prophylactic knee bracing in college football. *Am J Sports Med* 1987;15:111-116.

5. Grace TG, Skipper BJ, Newberry JC, Nelson MA, Sweetser ER, Rothman ML: Prophylactic knee braces and injury to the lower extremity. *J Bone Joint Surg Am* 1988;70:422-427.

6. Sitler M, Ryan J, Hopkinson W, et al: The efficacy of a prophylactic knee brace to reduce knee injuries in football: A prospective, randomized study at West Point. *Am J Sports Med* 1990;18:310-315.

7. Albright JP, Powell JW, Smith W, et al: Medial collateral ligament knee sprains in college football: Effectiveness of preventive braces. *Am J Sports Med* 1994;22:12-18.

8. Garrick JG, Requa RK: Prophylactic Knee Bracing. *Am J Sports Med* 1987;16(Suppl 1):S118-S123.

9. Brown TD, Van Hoeck JE, Brand RA: Laboratory evaluation of prophylactic knee brace performance under dynamic valgus loading using a surrogate leg model. *Clin Sports Med* 1990;9:751-762.

10. France EP, Paulos LE: In vitro assessment of prophylactic knee brace function. *Clin Sports Med* 1990;9:823-841.

11. Baker BE: The effect of bracing on the collateral ligaments of the knee. *Clin Sports Med* 1990;9:843-851.

12. Branch TP, Hunter RE: Functional analysis of anterior cruciate ligament braces. *Clin Sports Med* 1990;9:771-797.

13. Ryder SH, Johnson RJ, Beynnon BD, Ettlinger CF: Prevention of ACL injuries. *J Sport Rehabil* 1997;6:80-95.

14. Nemeth G, Lamontagne M, Tho KS, Eriksson E: Electromyographic activity in expert downhill skiers using functional knee braces after anterior cruciate ligament injuries. *Am J Sports Med* 1997;25:635-641.

Chapter 4

Hormonal Risk Factors

Laura J. Huston, MS
Edward M. Wojtys, MD

Introduction

Anterior cruciate ligament (ACL) injury rates differ by sex in several sports, with women experiencing two to eight times higher injury rates than men in the same sports.[1-5] These different injury rates suggest that sex-related factors contribute to the unique vulnerability of the female knee to ACL injury, and these factors need to be understood to devise effective preventive strategies. The possible role of hormones in predisposing female athletes to injury of the ACL has recently been actively investigated.[6-8] The purpose of this chapter is to review the literature on the basic physiology of the menstrual cycle; the interaction between levels of the female hormones estrogen, progesterone, and relaxin and ligament structure; and the possible association between these fluctuating hormone levels and the high rate of ACL injuries seen in female athletes.

Hormone Levels During the Menstrual Cycle

The menstrual cycle encompasses three phases—follicular, ovulatory, and luteal—during which estrogen, progesterone, and relaxin levels fluctuate[9,10] (Figs. 1 and 2). During the follicular phase, all hormone concentrations are very low. The ovulatory phase comprises the day of ovulation and the 4 days preceding it. This second phase is characterized by a midcycle surge in estrogen and luteinizing hormone (LH), with peak estrogen concentrations occurring 48 hours prior to ovulation. Once ovulation has occurred, the empty follicle becomes a corpus luteum, which persists for 14 days before the initiation of menstruation. This phase is known as the luteal phase and is characterized by a significant rise in progesterone levels secondary to the secretion of this hormone by the corpus luteum. Relaxin, on the other hand, is typically not detectable in circulation until early in the luteal phase and first becomes apparent about 6 to 8 days after the LH peak[11-14] (Fig. 2).

The normal menstrual cycle has a length of approximately 28 days. Variability in cycle length is mainly determined by the variable length of the follicular phase; the other phases are much more constant.[15]

Several methods are available to document cycle phase. The most common methods are by either serum or urine assay.[16] However, care must be

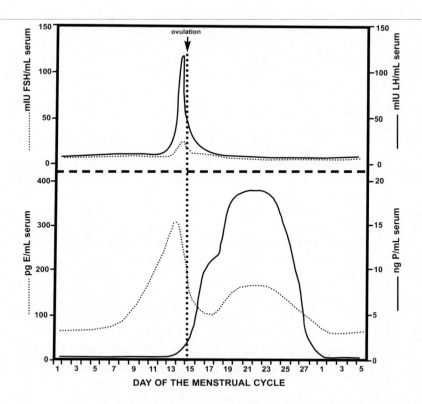

Fig. 1 *Serum concentrations of follicle-stimulating hormone (FSH), luteinizing hormone (LH), estrogen (E), and progesterone (P) through the menstrual cycle. (Reproduced with permission from Espey LL, Halim IAB: Characteristics and control of the normal menstrual cycle. Ob Gyn Clin North Am 1990;17:275–298.)*

taken when taking serum measurements, as the hormone levels are pulsatile. Monitoring the basal body temperature is also used to determine the mid-cycle estrogen surge, but this method is unreliable for the remainder of the cycle.

Existence of Hormone Receptors in Ligaments

The expression of estrogen and progesterone receptor proteins in target cells is a prerequisite for hormone action.[17] Estrogen and progesterone receptor sites have been reported in human ACL cells, suggesting that female sex hormones may play a role in the structure and composition of the ACL.[18,19] In addition, Galey and associates[20] recently discovered that relaxin receptor sites exist in the ACL.

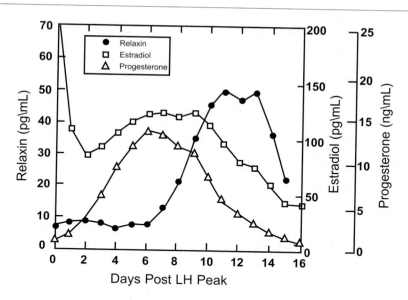

Fig. 2 *Mean serum concentrations of relaxin, estradiol, and progesterone during a normal menstrual cycle. Undetectable levels were given the value of 10 ng/L when calculating the means. The detection limit of the assay is 20 ng/L. (Reproduced with permission from Stewart DR, Nakajima ST, Overstreet JW, Boyers SP, Lasley BL: Relaxin as a biomarker for human pregnancy, in MacLenna AH, Tregear GW, Bryant-Greenwood GD (eds): Progress in Relaxin Research: 2nd International Congress on the Hormone Relaxin. River Edge, NJ, World Scientific Publishers, 1994, pp 214-224.)*

Effects of Hormones

Cellular Mechanisms

Collagen, which is produced by fibroblasts, performs the major load-bearing function of the ACL.[21] Alterations in the metabolism of these collagen fibroblasts directly influence the quantity, type, and stability of the collagen in the ACL.[22]

It has been reported that with increasing levels of estrogen, both collagen synthesis and fibroblast proliferation significantly decrease.[23,24] In 1976, Hama and associates[25] investigated the effects of estrogen levels in the rat model. They found that increasing levels of estrogen decreased collagen content and fibril diameter in the rat hip joint. Shikata and associates[26] also reported that estrogen levels significantly affect the cellular makeup of collagen. Using a rat model, they found that estrogen increased the elastin content, fiber diameter, and the ratio of central elastin to peripheral microfibrils.

Collagen synthesis also decreases with increasing levels of relaxin.[27-29] Relaxin is responsible for the remodeling of the connective tissues of the pubic symphysis in pregnant mammals.[30] At the ultrastructural level, as the level of relaxin increases, dense collagen fibers are dissociated into smaller, more disorganized fibrils.[31] These relaxin-induced collagen bundles are less abundant, less ordered, and smaller in diameter. Thus, the expansion of the pubic ligament occurs via a decrease in the density and integrity of collagen bundles.[2] Interestingly, the effects of relaxin are enhanced by the presence of estrogen, while progesterone acts as an antagonist to both estrogen and relaxin.[27]

Mechanical Properties of Ligaments

Controversy exists as to whether hormone fluctuations associated with the menstrual cycle influence the mechanical properties of ligaments. Female sex hormones have been found to influence the binding forces within the fibers of connective tissue and thereby may affect the mechanical properties of ligaments.[32-36] Several studies have reported that estrogen and relaxin levels affect the mechanical properties of ligaments. For example, Levine[37] demonstrated a dose-dependent response between estrogen and relaxin and ligament stiffness and laxity in the mouse model; increasing levels of estrogen plus relaxin led to greater ligament stiffness values. Slauterbeck and associates[38] reported that the administration of estrogen significantly reduced the tensile properties of rabbit ACL. However, these results must be interpreted cautiously because many of the studies involve the administration of hormone concentrations that are not physiologic (eg, levels seen during pregnancy or other superphysiologic levels). Recently, Strickland and associates[39] investigated the mechanical properties of sheep ligaments, using physiologic doses of estrogen. They found no effect on estrogen level concentrations or change in mechanical properties of the ACL or medial cruciate ligament. Similarly, Belanger and associates[40] found no correlation between ACL tensile strength and serum estrogen levels in rats.

Effect of Oral Contraceptives

The steroids contained in oral contraceptives (OCs) are known to significantly affect the hormonal cycle, mainly through suppression of the pituitary. The synthetic steroids in OCs have estrogenic and progestogenic effects, which inhibit follicle stimulating hormone (FSH) and LH production by the pituitary by means of negative feedback. OCs also induce some change in the secretion of relaxin.[41] Follicular growth, ovulation, and production of a corpus luteum is thus prevented.

When looking at the effect of OCs, it is important to distinguish between monophasic preparations, in which the doses of estrogen and progesterone remain constant throughout the pill cycle, and multiphasic preparations, in which the doses are varied over the cycle to mimic normal physiologic values of estrogen and progesterone. Multiphasic preparations generally contain lower doses of progesterone than do monophasic preparations.

If hormonal fluctuations during the menstrual cycle may influence the risk of injury during sporting activities, it is reasonable to ask whether OCs, by means of their effects on the hormonal cycle, affect physical performance and the risk for sports injuries. Furthermore, OCs may influence other variables important for physical performance, such as joint laxity and neuromuscular coordination. There is only one study to date looking at the association between knee injuries and OC use. In a prospective study, Möller-Nielsen and Hammar[42] monitored 86 young soccer players throughout 1,008 menstrual cycles. They found that women on OCs had fewer traumatic injuries than women not on OCs ($P < 0.01$). However, additional research needs to be done to confirm these findings.

Association Between Hormone Levels and ACL Injury

Several investigators have attempted to link hormone fluctuations during the menstrual cycle to the rate of ACL injuries, but with conflicting results. In 1998, Wojtys and associates[8] reported more injuries than expected while patients were in the ovulatory phase of the menstrual cycle (days 10 through 14, when estrogen levels surge), while fewer injuries occurred while patients were in the follicular phase (days 1 through 9, when estrogen and progesterone levels are low). Also in 1998, Myklebust and associates[7] found that significantly fewer injuries occurred during the midcycle estrogen surge (days 8 through 14) in a group of Norwegian team handball players. The significant difference between these two studies may be the patient populations studied. The study by Wojtys and associates examined women with regular menstrual cycles who were not taking OCs, while half of the subjects in the study by Myklebust and associates were taking OCs. In 1989, Möller-Nielsen had linked OC use to lower injury rates in women; however, these injury rates were classified only as general traumatic injuries and did not isolate knee or ACL injuries. A 1998-1999 survey of 103 ACL-injured female National Collegiate Athletic Association basketball players found that athletes tended to be injured just before or after the onset of menses, regardless of their use of OCs.[2]

Conclusion

Results of studies so far regarding the interaction between female hormone concentrations and compositional changes in the ACL are compelling. However, a consensus is lacking regarding the association of menstrual cycle phase with the incidence of ACL injuries. More rigorous studies need to be performed before treatment or prevention recommendations can be made.

Fast Facts

Fact: Estrogen and progesterone receptor sites have been reported in human ACL cells, suggesting that female sex hormones may play a role in the structure and composition of the ACL.

Fact: With increasing levels of estrogen, collagen synthesis and fibroblast proliferation significantly decrease.

Fact: Collagen synthesis also decreases with increasing levels of relaxin.

Fact: Controversy exists as to whether hormone fluctuations associated with the menstrual cycle influence the mechanical properties of ligaments.

Caution: Data linking ACL injury to hormone levels, as indirectly inferred from injury occurrence during the monthly menstrual cycle, are inconsistent.

Caution: Insufficient evidence exists to suggest altering hormone levels to prevent injury.

Caution: Insufficient evidence exists to suggest that restricting women from sports participation during any portion of the menstrual cycle would prevent injury.

References

1.   Arendt E, Dick R: Knee injury patterns among men and women in collegiate basketball and soccer: NCAA data and review of literature. *Am J Sports Med* 1995;23:694-701.

2.   Arendt EA, Agel J, Dick R: Anterior cruciate ligament injury patterns among collegiate men and women. *Athletic Training* 1999;24:86-92.

3.   Lindenfeld TN, Schmitt DJ, Hendy MP, Mangine RE, Noyes FR: Incidence of injury in indoor soccer. *Am J Sports Med* 1994;22:364-371.

4.   Malone TR, Hardaker WT, Garrett WE, et al: Relationship of gender to anterior cruciate ligament injuries in intercollegiate basketball players. *J South Orthop Assoc* 1993;2:36-39.

5.   Harmon KG, Ireland ML: Gender differences in noncontact anterior cruciate ligament injuries. *Clin Sports Med* 2000;19:287-302.

6.   Möller-Nielsen J, Hammar M: Sports injuries and oral contraceptive use: Is there a relationship? *Sports Med* 1991;12:152-160.

7.   Myklebust G, Maehlum S, Holm I, Bahr R: A prospective cohort study of anterior cruciate ligament injuries in elite Norwegian team handball. *Scand J Med Sci Sports* 1998;8:149-153.

8.   Wojtys EM, Huston LJ, Lindenfeld TN, Hewett TE, Greenfield ML: Association between the menstrual cycle and anterior cruciate ligament injuries in female athletes. *Am J Sports Med* 1998;26:614-619.

9.   Owen JA Jr: Physiology of the menstrual cycle. *Am J Clin Nutr* 1975;28:333-338.

10. Speroff L, Glass RH, Kase NG: Regulation of the menstrual cycle, in Speroff L, Glass RH, Kase NG (eds): *Clinical Gynecologic Endocrinology and Infertility,* ed 2. Baltimore, MD, Williams & Wilkins, 1978, pp 49-63.

11. Stewart DR, Nakajima ST, Overstreet JW, Boyers SO, Lasley BL: Relaxin as a biomarker for human pregnancy detection, in MacLennan AM, Tregear GW, Bryant-Greenwood GD (eds): *Progress in Relaxin Research: 2nd International Congress on the Hormone Relaxin,* River Edge, NJ, Global Publications Services, 1994, pp 199-213.

12. Johnson MR, Carter G, Grint C, Lightman SL: Relationship between ovarian steroids, gonadotrophins and relaxin during the menstrual cycle. *Acta Endocrinol* (Copenh) 1993;129:121-125.

13. Weiss G: Relaxin. *Clin Perinatol* 1983;10:641-651.

14. Weiss G: Relaxin levels in the human, in MacLennan AM, Tregear GW, Bryant-Greenwood GD (eds): *Progress in Relaxin Research: 2nd International Congress on the Hormone Relaxin,* River Edge, NJ, Global Publications Services, 1994, pp 199-213.

15. Vollman RF: The Menstrual Cycle: *Major Problems in Obstetrics and Gynecology.* Philadelphia, PA, WB Saunders, 1977, Vol. 7.

16. Landgren BM, Unden AL, Diczfalusy E: Hormonal profile of the cycle in 68 normally menstruating women. *Acta Endocrinol* 1980;94:89-98.

17. Jensen EV, Greene GL, Closs LE, DeSombre ER, Nadji M: Receptors reconsidered: A 20-year perspective. *Recent Prog Horm Res* 1982;38:1-40.

18. Liu SH, al-Shaikh R, Panossian V, et al: Primary immunolocalization of estrogen and progesterone target cells in the human anterior cruciate ligament. *J Orthop Res* 1996;14:526-533.

19. Sciore P, Frank CB, Hart DA: Identification of sex hormone receptors in human and rabbit ligaments of the knee by reverse transcription-polymerase chain reaction: Evidence that receptors are present in tissue from both male and female subjects. *J Orthop Res* 1998;16:604-610.

20. Galey S, Arnold C, Konieczko E, Cooney T: Immunohistochemical identification of relaxin receptors on anterior cruciate ligaments. *Trans Orthop Res Soc* 2000;25:794.

21. Smith BA, Livesay GA, Woo SL: Biology and biomechanics of the anterior cruciate ligament. *Clin Sports Med* 1993;12:637-670.

22. Burgeson RE, Nimni ME: Collagen types: Molecular structure and tissue distribution. *Clin Orthop* 1992;282:250-272.

23. Liu SH, al-Shaikh RA, Panossian V, Finerman GA, Lane JM: Estrogen affects the cellular metabolism of the anterior cruciate ligament. *Am J Sports Med* 1997;25:704-709.

24. Yu WD, Liu SH, Hatch JD, Panossian V, Finerman GA: Effect of estrogen on cellular metabolism of the human anterior cruciate ligament. *Clin Orthop* 1999;366:229-238.

25. Hama H, Yamamuro T, Takeda T: Experimental studies on connective tissue of the capsular ligament: Influences of aging and sex hormones. *Acta Orthop Scand* 1976;47:473-479.

26. Shikata J, Sanada H, Tamamuro T, Takeda T: Experimental studies of the elastic fiber of the capsular ligament: Influence of aging and sex hormones on the hip joint capsule of rats. *Connect Tissue Res* 1979;7:21-27.

27. Samuel CS, Butkus A, Coghlan JP, Bateman JF: The effect of relaxin on collagen metabolism in the nonpregnant rat pubic symphysis: The influence of estrogen and progesterone in regulating relaxin activity. *Endocrinology* 1996;137:3884-3890.

28. Unemori EN, Amento EP: Relaxin modulates synthesis and secretion of procollagenase and collagen by human dermal fibroblasts. *J Biol Chem* 1990;265:10681-10685.

29. Unemori EN, Beck LS, Lee WP, et al: Human relaxin decreases collagen accumulation in vivo in two rodent models of fibrosis. *J Invest Dermatol* 1993;101:280-285.

30. Goldsmith LT, Weiss G, Steinetz BG: Relaxin and its role in pregnancy. *Endocrinol Metab Clin North Am* 1995;24:171-186.

31. McDonald JK, Schwabe C: Relaxin-induced elevations of cathepsin B and dipeptidyl peptidase I in the mouse pubic symphysis, with localization by fluorescence enzyme histochemistry. *Ann NY Acad Sci* 1982;380:178-186.

32. Booth FW, Tipton CM: Ligamentous strength measurements in pre-pubescent and pubescent rats. *Growth* 1970;34:177-185.

33. Calguneri M, Bird HA, Wright V: Changes in joint laxity occurring during pregnancy. *Ann Rheum Dis* 1982;41:126-128.

34. Cheah SH, Ng KH, Johgalingam VT, Ragavan M: The effects of oestradiol and relaxin on extensibility and collagen organisation of the pregnant rat cervix. *J Endocrinol* 1995;146:331-337.

35. Dyer RF, Sodek J, Heersche JN: The effect of 17 beta-estradiol on collagen and noncollagenous protein synthesis in the uterus and some periodontal tissues. *Endocrinology* 1980;107:1014-1021.

36. Wood M, Luthin B, Lester G, Dahners L: Creep in tendons is potentiated by a pentapeptide (NKISK) and by relaxin which produce collagen fiber sliding. *Trans Orthop Res Soc* 2000;25:61.

37. Levine RE, Steinetz BG, Hannafin JA, Granda SM, Wright TM: Mechanical response to the interpubic ligament and knee joint in mice to relaxin. *Orthop Trans* 1999;24:328.

38. Slauterbeck J, Clevenger C, Lundberg W, Burchfield DM: Estrogen level alters the failure load of the rabbit anterior cruciate ligament. *J Orthop Res* 1999;17:405-408.

39. Strickland SM, Belknap TW, Levine RE, Turner AS, Wright TM, Hannafin JA: Lack of hormonal influences on mechanical properties of sheep knee ligaments. *Trans Orthop Res Soc* 2000;25:21.

40. Belanger M, Moore DC, McAllister SC, Ehrlich MG: The mechanical properties of rat ACL are independent of serum estrogen level. *Trans Orthop Res Soc* 2000;25:151.

41. Wreje U, Kristiansson P, Aberg H, Bystrom B, von Schoultz B: Serum levels of relaxin during the menstrual cycle and oral contraceptive use. *Gynecol Obstet Invest* 1995;39:197-200.

42. Möller-Nielsen J, Hammar M: Women's soccer injuries in relation to the menstrual cycle and oral contraceptive use. *Med Sci Sports Exerc* 1989;21:126-129.

Chapter 5
Anatomic Risk Factors

Mary Lloyd Ireland, MD

Potential Anatomic Risk Factors

Various anatomic differences between men and women have been implicated as risk factors for noncontact anterior cruciate ligament (ACL) injury. They have been touted as responsible for the increased rate of noncontact ACL injuries in women. When compared with men of equal age, women are more likely to have less muscle mass per total body weight, greater joint hyperextension, greater physiologic rotational laxity, increased femoral internal rotation and anteversion, genu valgus, a greater Q angle, tibial external rotation, forefoot pronation, and pes planus, as well as a smaller ACL housed in a smaller femoral notch[1-5] (Fig. 1, *A* and *B*). In addition, differences in skeletal size between men and women have been reported. Powers[1] reported that women have a smaller distal femur, proximal tibia, and patella than men of comparable size. Gilsanz[2] compared sizes of axial and appendicular skeletons and noted that vertebral bodies in women were smaller than those in men. Horton and Hall[3] reported that women have shorter femurs than men, but that men have greater absolute pelvic width.

Conflicting statements have been made regarding the center of gravity in men and women. In late childhood and adolescence, the ratio of upper body length to lower body length shows little difference by sex (0.98 in boys and 0.99 in girls).[4,5] The lower extremity is not significantly longer in boys than in girls. Similarly, Atwater[6] described only small differences in the center of gravity between men and women, whereas others attribute women's increased balance stability to their lower center of gravity.[5]

Women are more likely to have an anteriorly rotated pelvis.[7] In the anteriorly rotated pelvic position, the hip is in internal rotation and varus, and the knee is in valgus recurvatum. The tibia is externally rotated, the forefoot is pronated, and the lumbar lordosis is increased. There is extension of the thoracolumbar spine.

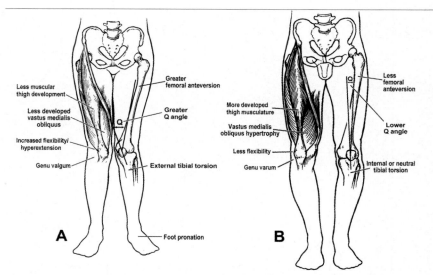

Fig. 1 *Female (A) and male (B) lower extremity alignment. Women have greater femoral anteversion and Q angle, increased flexibility, less developed musculature, less developed vastus medialis obliquus, narrower femoral notch, a tendency toward genu valgum, and external tibial torsion. Men have less femoral anteversion and a smaller Q angle, more developed thigh musculature, vastus medialis obliquus hypertrophy, less flexibility, wider femoral notch, tendency toward genu varum, and internal or neutral tibial torsion. (Reproduced with permission from Fu FH, Stone DA (eds):* Sports Injuries: Mechanism, Prevention, and Treatment, *ed 2. Baltimore, MD, Williams & Wilkins, 1994, p 154.)*

The Significance of Anatomic Factors

The various anatomic differences between men and women have not been proven to explain higher noncontact ACL injury rates in women. At present, there are no studies conclusively relating static or dynamic anatomic factors to ACL injury. One lower extremity alignment study done by Meister and associates[8] comparing ACL-injured patients to non-ACL-injured patients found no statistical difference in the femoral anteversion or Q angle between the two groups. The authors felt that there was a statistical difference in the thigh-foot angle, with the injured group measuring $21.6° \pm 6.8°$ and the uninjured group measuring $18.3° \pm 4.4°$. This preliminary study has not been verified. More studies are needed to clarify the influence of anatomic factors on ACL injury rates.

Fast Facts

Fact: There are anatomic variations in lower extremity size and alignment between men and women.

Fact: To date, no anatomic variation, static or dynamic has been conclusively associated with an increased risk for ACL injury.

Caution: Based on our present knowledge, no athlete should be considered at higher risk for ACL injury and therefore excluded from sport participation on the basis of skeletal size or structure, or overall limb alignment.

References

1. Powers JA: Characteristic features of injuries in the knee in women. *Clin Orthop* 1979;143:120-124.

2. Gilsanz V, Boechat MI, Gilsanz R, Loro ML, Roe TF, Goodman WG: Gender differences in vertebral sizes in adults: Biomechanical implications. *Radiology* 1994;190:678-682.

3. Horton MG, Hall TL: Quadriceps femoris muscle angle: Normal values and relationships with gender and selected skeletal measures. *Phys Ther* 1989;69:897-901.

4. Tachdjian MO (ed): *Pediatric Orthopedics*, Vol 1. Philadelphia, PA, WB Saunders, 1990.

5. Arendt EA: Orthopaedic issues for active and athletic women. *Clin Sports Med* 1994;13:483-503.

6. Atwater AE: Biomechanics and the female athlete, in Puhl JL, Brown CH, Voy RO (eds): *Sports Science Perspectives for Women*. Champaign, IL, Human Kinetics, 1988, pp 1-12.

7. Hruska R: Pelvic stability influences lower-extremity kinematics. *Biomechanics* 1998;5:23-29.

8. Meister K, Huegel MO, Rolle GA, Indelicato PA, Horodyski MB: Abstract: The influence of rotational alignment of the lower extremity on noncontact injuries to the anterior cruciate ligament in the female athlete. *65th Annual Meeting Proceedings*. Rosemont, IL, American Academy of Orthopaedic Surgeons, 1998, p 79.

Chapter 6

Relationship Between Notch Width Index and Risk of Noncontact ACL Injury

Elizabeth A. Arendt, MD

Introduction

The literature is replete with articles exploring a possible relationship between the width of the intercondylar notch and the risk of injuring the anterior cruciate ligament (ACL) (Table 1). This idea was originally explored with regard to bilateral ACL injury. Further investigations looked at unilateral ACL injuries and, more recently, whether a gender difference exists with regard to notch width index.

The term notch width index (NWI) was coined by Souryal and associates.[4] The NWI is a measurement made from a notch view radiograph (position: prone bent knee). LaPrade and Burnett[10] (1994) have written the only article that discusses rigorously the technique used to take this radiograph. They state that "no measurement differences were found between notch radiographs for each subject when a template was used to control leg rotation and knee flexion, but there was a statistical difference when these were compared to radiographs where the template was not used." Additionally, there were significant differences in recorded notch widths when the leg was rotated more than 15° (personal communication). Because the NWI involves small numbers and a ratio, 1 mm difference in the radiographic measurement can make a difference in the statistical analysis.

Literature Review

The two largest population studies, Souryal and Freeman[7] and LaPrade and Burnett,[10] both used this standard notch view. Again, only LaPrade and Burnett controlled leg rotation and knee flexion using a template. Souryal and Freeman measured 907 high school athletes (783 were included in the study) from various schools. Although the same view was used, it is unlikely that the technique was rigorously controlled. The results differ, with Souryal and Freeman finding the NWI smaller in women than in men in the noninjured population. LaPrade and Burnett found no such relationship. Souryal's total population (783) was larger than LaPrade's (213). Souryal and Freeman estimated the number of women in their study to be one third

**Table 1 Summary of Literature Regarding Notch Width Index
and ACL Injuries***

Reference	Population	Measurement Technique
Mensch and Amstutz[1] 1975	30 cadaver knees, mean age 73 F = 16, M = 14 53 radiograph knees, mean age 38 F = 23, M = 30	Cadaver: Direct caliper measurement Radiograph: AP standing, notch
Anderson et al[2] 1987	14 bilateral ACL injuries (Group 1) 17 unilateral injuries (Group 2) 17 with no known knee injuries (Group 3) Mean age = 25 Retrospective study	CT scan Direct measurement
Houseworth et al[3] 1987	Patients with acute ACL injury and no known knee injury 100 patients, 50 in each group Retrospective study	Computer graphic study Notch radiographic view with computer graphic analysis
Souryal et al[4] 1988	Bilateral ACL injuries (Group 1) Acute ACL injuries (Group 2) Normal knees (Group 3) Mean age = 19 N = 50 for each group Retrospective study	Notch radiographic view Defines NWI as ratio of width of ICN to width of femoral condyle, using radiographic landmarks
Good et al[5] 1991	93 chronic ACL (Group 1) 62 acute ACL (Group 2) 38 cadavers (Group 3) Intraoperative measurements and cadaver study	Direct measurement of anterior notch opening using a caliper technique
Schickendantz and Weiker[6] 1993	30 unilateral injuries (Group 1) 31 bilateral injuries (Group 2) 30 normal knees (Group 3) Mean age = 23.5 years Retrospective study	Used eight different mathematical measurement ratios from standing notch radiographic view and direct measurement Radiograph: Standing notch view
Souryal and Freeman[7] 1993	783 high school athletes Mean age = 16 years Numbers of men and women are not given Prospective study	Notch radiographic view, measured NWI No radiographic template was used

*F = female; M = male; NW = notch width
NC-ACL= noncontact anterior cruciate ligament; LFC = lateral femoral condyle;
NWI = notch width index; ICN = intercondylar notch
† Not Souryal's view

Conclusion	Difference by Sex
NWI symmetric between right and left knee NWI (normal) = NWI (NC-ACL)	F NWI < M NWI not significant ($P = 0.10$) F = 40, M = 40
Mean NWI: F = 0.243, M = 0.258	
Mean NW (direct measurement) F = 13.9 mm, M = 15.9 mm Female NW < male NW with height and weight as covariants	

Statements Supported by the Literature

Radiographic Notch Measurements

Despite the limitations in the various radiographic techniques and the possible lack of controlling for rotation, the literature supports the following general statements:

1. Notch width (regardless of measurement technique) of bilateral ACL-injured knees is smaller than that of unilateral ACL-injured knees.

2. Notch width of bilateral and unilateral ACL-injured knees is smaller than the notch width of normal controls.

3. Grouping study populations by sex shows that the width of women's notches is smaller than the width of men's notches.

4. Arranging study populations by sex shows that the NWI (relation of condylar width to notch width) in women is smaller than the NWI in men.

5. A relationship exists between the width of the bicondylar femur and the width of the notch. The smaller the femur, the smaller the notch.

Statement 4 may need clarification. Shelbourne and associates[13,15] report that women have smaller notches than men of similar height. However, women appear to have a smaller bicondylar width than men of the same height, and the bicondylar width appears to be correlated to the width of the notch, even in Shelbourne and associates' study. Shelbourne and associates correlate the height of the patient (not the height of the femur or the width of the bicondylar femur) to the notch width. Therefore, the literature is consistent in that the width of the bicondylar femur is related to the width of the notch.

Intraoperative Notch Measurements

Intraoperative measurements seem to produce less agreement. Shelbourne and associates'[13,15] direct measurements are quite small (women, 13.9 mm; men, 15.9 mm). These are significantly smaller than Good and associates'[5] measurements, which also involved an intraoperative caliper measurement. Good and associates' smallest measurement is 16.1 mm, in the chronic ACL-deficient knee; knees with acute ACL tears averaged 18.1 mm, and cadaver knees averaged 20.4 mm. Additionally, an earlier cadaver study by Mensch and Amstutz[1] gives a mean notch width of 18.7 mm in women and 20.8 mm in men. This measurement was arrived at by looking at parameters for a total knee arthroplasty, however, and may not be representative of the population discussed here. Nonetheless, the values found by the direct measurement techniques of Shelbourne and associates (13.9 mm to 15.9 mm) are considerably smaller than others stated in the literature.

What Is Not Known

Mechanism of Injury

If one concludes that the size of the intercondylar notch is related to risk of ACL injury, the question still remains as to how notch size contributes to the ACL injury. Munetta and associates[12] suggest that patients with small notches have normal-size ACLs and that impingement contributes to the tear. Others believe that a small intercondylar notch houses a small ACL. Shelbourne and associates[13] state that "the size of the ACL and not the notch size itself is more important in determining the likelihood of sustaining an ACL tear." However, this has not been conclusively shown. Arendt and associates (American Orthopaedic Society for Sports Medicine, summer meeting, Orlando, Florida, 1995) looked at the size of the notch versus the size of the ACL using magnetic resonance imaging (MRI) of normal knees, and found that it was difficult to measure consistently the ACL size in a single transverse MRI plane because of the two-bundle nature of the ACL and the fact that it rotates. The difficulty of measuring the ACL in a single plane is confirmed by Harner and associates,[8] who found that the cross-sectional shapes of the posterior cruciate ligament and the ACL are irregular and vary between the femoral and tibial insertion. They also found that the cross-sectional shape of the ligaments changes with knee flexion. Therefore, a single measurement on a single radiographic view is unlikely to be representative of the size of the ACL.

Therefore, the exact role that a small notch plays in creating an ACL tear remains speculative. Does a small notch create increased stress on the ACL in certain positions, particularly knee internal rotation and hyperextension? If so, do knee positions that create "ACL impingement" correspond to known knee positions during ACL injury? Does a small notch house a small ACL with concomitant decrease in ligament strength, thus being susceptible to injury from the stress of a pounding or pivoting sport?

Relation of NWI to Sex

In the prospective study by Souryal and Freeman,[7] the distribution of NWIs in male and female athletes approaches a bell-shaped curve. In addition, Souryal and Freeman's study, measuring 783 athletes, found female athletes' NWIs to be smaller than those in male athletes in the noninjured population. LaPrade and Burnett[10] found no such relation in their study population base of 213. It is difficult to know if the difference is so small that a larger population base is needed to statistically uncover the difference. Another confounding feature is that LaPrade and Burnett controlled the rotation, as stated previously, and perhaps their numbers are therefore more accurate.

What is not known about this particular distribution of athletes is whether the shorter women sustaining these injuries were disproportionately weighted into sports that are known to have a high risk of ACL injuries. In other words, if most runners and volleyball players are tall and most gymnasts and soccer players are short, this might result in a disproportionate number of noncontact ACL injuries occurring in smaller female athletes. The same could be said about the smaller male athlete. Therefore, it would be interesting to look at a population of athletes in sports that are known to put the participants at high risk for ACL injuries, eg, soccer and basketball. Examining a prospective NWI profile to see if the smaller notch puts the athlete at a higher risk of injury would be helpful in determining the relationship between sex, notch width, and ACL injury.

What can we conclude about people with small NWIs who do not sustain an ACL injury? Shelbourne and associates' 1997 article[13] reports a smaller NWI in women than men. However, although 66% of the female controls had NWIs less than or equal to 15 mm, and 34% of the male controls had NWIs less than or equal to 15 mm, these "athletic" young adults did not sustain an ACL injury. However, their specific athletic activities were not mentioned.

Implications for Prevention

If a strong correlation between a small NWI and a high risk for noncontact ACL injury becomes apparent, it begs the question: Can anything be done about it? If the mechanism of ACL injury in knees with small notches was known, potential prevention strategies could be developed. If it is a mechanical situation, one might still be able to control knee rotation prophylactically through muscle strengthening or avoiding positions of risk. If risk of injury is purely related to the strength of the ACL, risk modification would be difficult. However, from a teleologic standpoint, it would seem unusual for a small person to be disadvantaged by having a small ACL when typically the structures of the human body have strength and size appropriate to body build.

Summary

In reviewing the literature, I found 15 papers on the relationship of NWIs to ACL injuries. The population samples range from 20 female athletes to 783 high school athletes. Differences by sex were addressed in some manner in 9 of the 15 studies.

The research varies considerably with regard to population group studied (cadaver, bilateral ACL tear, acute or chronic ACL tear), measurement technique used (radiographic measurement, computed tomography, direct intraoperative or cadaver measurement, computer graphics), and whether the absolute notch width or the NWI is measured. Because of this variability in the literature, it is not possible to make definitive statements concerning size of the ACL and notch width parameters. Also, the measurement technique varies too much to make definitive statements concerning the relationship of the size of the notch to the risk of a unilateral ACL injury.

Recommendations

A prospective study of the relationship of NWI to ACL injury in both men and women is imperative. The measurement technique should be standardized and controlled for internal and external measurement errors. The population-based study should examine similar sports or activity levels for both men and women. The study population should include a population known to be at high risk for noncontact ACL injury. Ideally, the mechanism of noncontact ACL injury should be recorded to try to correlate the relationship between the biomechanical variables of ACL injury and the anatomic variables of notch and ACL size.

Fast Facts

Fact: The femoral notch width of bilateral ACL-injured knees is less than unilateral ACL-injured knees, which is less than normal controls.

Fact: The width of the notch in women is less than the width of the notch in men.

Fact: The smaller the condylar width of the femur, the smaller the notch.

Fact: Femoral rotation can influence notch width.

Caution: Data are insufficient to recommend exclusion of an athlete from sport based on notch size.

Caution: Evidence is insufficient to firmly establish a relationship between sex, notch width, ACL size, and noncontact ACL injuries.

References

1. Mensch JS, Amstutz HC: Knee morphology as a guide to knee replacement. *Clin Orthop* 1975;112:231-241.

2. Anderson AF, Lipscomb AB, Liudahl KJ, Addlestone RB: Analysis of the intercondylar notch by computed tomography. *Am J Sports Med* 1987;15:547-552.

3. Houseworth SW, Mauro VJ, Mellon BA, Kieffer DA: The intercondylar notch in acute tears of the anterior cruciate ligament: A computer graphics study. *Am J Sports Med* 1987;15:221-224.

4. Souryal TO, Moore HA, Evans JP: Bilaterality in anterior cruciate ligament injuries: Associated intercondylar notch stenosis. *Am J Sports Med* 1988;16:449-454.

5. Good L, Odensten M, Gillquist J: Intercondylar notch measurements with special reference to anterior cruciate ligament surgery. *Clin Orthop* 1991;263:185-189.

6. Schickendantz MS, Weiker GG: The predictive value of radiographs in the evaluation of unilateral and bilateral anterior cruciate ligament injuries. *Am J Sports Med* 1993;21:110-113.

7. Souryal TO, Freeman TR: Intercondylar notch size and anterior cruciate ligament injuries in athletes: A prospective study. *Am J Sports Med* 1993;21:535-539.

8. Harner CD, Paulos LE, Greenwald AE, Rosenberg TD, Cooley VC: Detailed analysis of patients with bilateral anterior cruciate ligament injuries. *Am J Sports Med* 1994;22:37-43.

9. Herzog RJ, Silliman JF, Hutton K, Rodkey WG, Steadman JR: Measurements of the intercondylar notch by plain film radiography and magnetic resonance imaging. *Am J Sports Med* 1994;22:204-210.

10. LaPrade RF, Burnett QM II: Femoral intercondylar notch stenosis and correlation to anterior cruciate ligament injuries: A prospective study. *Am J Sports Med* 1994;22:198-203.

11. Lund-Hanssen H, Gannon J, Engebretsen L, Holen KJ, Anda S, Vatten L: Intercondylar notch width and the risk for anterior cruciate ligament rupture: A case control study in 46 female handball players. *Acta Orthop Scand* 1994;65:529-532.

12. Muneta T, Takakuda K, Yamamoto H: Intercondylar notch width and its relation to the configuration and cross-sectional area of the anterior cruciate ligament: A cadaveric knee study. *Am J Sports Med* 1997;25:69-72.

13. Shelbourne KD, Facibene WA, Hunt JJ: Radiographic and intraoperative intercondylar notch width measurements in men and women with unilateral and bilateral anterior cruciate ligament tears. *Knee Surg Sports Traumatol Arthrosc* 1997;5:229-233.

14. Teitz CC, Lind BK, Sacks BM: Symmetry of the femoral notch width index. *Am J Sports Med* 1997;25:687-690.

15. Shelbourne KD, Davis TJ, Klootwyk TE: The relationship between intercondylar notch width of the femur and the incidence of anterior cruciate ligament tears: A prospective study. *Am J Sports Med* 1998;26:402-408.

Chapter 7

The Role of Mechanoreceptors in Functional Joint Stability

Scott M. Lephart, PhD, ATC
Bryan L. Riemann, MA, ATC

The term "functional joint stability" (FJS) refers to the joint stability required for normal performance during functional activity. The complementary relationships between the static and dynamic components of a joint contribute to FJS, with the level of contribution from each component varying with the individual and the task. The dynamic contributions emerge from precise neuromotor control over the skeletal muscles crossing the joint. Skeletal muscle activation may be initiated consciously, directly from voluntary command, or unconsciously and automatically, as part of a motor program or in response to sensory stimuli.

Neuromuscular Control and Proprioception

Regardless of the source of muscle activation, accurate sensory information concerning the external and internal environmental conditions is required to tailor the specifics of the activation sequence to respective conditional demands (Fig. 1). The term "neuromuscular control" refers to unconscious activation of the dynamic restraints surrounding a joint in response to sensory stimuli. According to Matthews[1] and recent interpretations by Lephart and associates (Ref. 2 and unpublished data, 2000), Sherrington[3,4] described proprioception as the afferent information arising from the periphery concerning regulation of postural equilibrium, joint stability, and several conscious peripheral sensations.

Proprioception is the sensory source best suited for providing the information necessary for mediating neuromuscular control, thereby enhancing FJS. Sources of proprioceptive information include mechanoreceptors, located in muscle, articular, and cutaneous tissues, that are responsible for transducing mechanical events occurring in their respective tissues into neural signals. The neural information provided by these receptors is conveyed via afferent neurons to the spinal cord. Upon arrival at the spinal cord, many of the afferent neurons bifurcate, with the projections synapsing directly with gamma motoneurons (γ-MNs), alpha motoneurons (α-MNs), or interneurons. Many of the interneurons provide the basis for sensory inte-

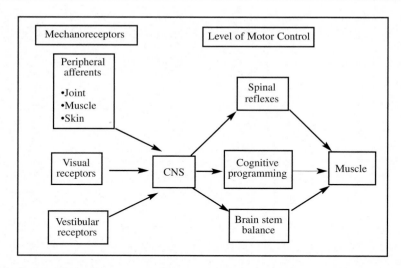

Fig. 1 Neuromuscular control pathways. Reproduced with permission from Lephart S, Fu F (eds): Proprioception and Lephart S, Fu F (eds) : Proprioception and Neuromuscular Control in Joint Stability. *Champaign, IL Human Kinetics, 2000*

gration and motor control at the spinal level, while others form the ascending tracts leading to higher central nervous system (CNS) structures (Fig. 2).

The Role of the Cerebellum

The spinocerebellar pathways leading to the cerebellum more than likely provide the organizational core of supraspinal control over the dynamic restraints. Working entirely subconsciously, the cerebellum has an essential role in planning and modifying motor activities by comparing the intended movement with the outcome movement.[5] Continual inflows of information from the motor control areas and central and peripheral sensory areas provide the means by which the cerebellum can accomplish this task.

The cerebellum is divided into three functional areas (Table 1). The first division, the vestibulocerebellum, is mostly responsible for controlling the axial muscles, which are involved with postural equilibrium. The second division, the cerebrocerebellum, is mainly involved with the planning and initiation of movements, especially those requiring precise and rapid dexterous limb motion.[5] The third division, the spinocerebellum, receives afferent information from the somatosensory, visual, and vestibular systems and adjusts ongoing movements through influential corrections with the brain stem and motor cortex. The spinocerebellum also uses somatosensory inputs for the feedback regulation of muscle tone through regulation of static γ-MN drive to the muscle spindles.[5]

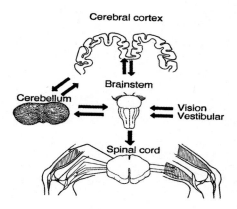

Fig. 2 The role of proprioception in mediating neuromuscular control of joint stability. (Reproduced with permission from Lephart S, Fu F (eds): Proprioception and Neuromuscular Control in Joint Stability. *Champaign, IL, Human Kinetics, 2000.)*

Table 1 The Three Functional Areas of the Cerebellum

Vestibulocerebellum	Primarily controls axial muscles involved with postural equilibrium.
Cerebrocerebellum	Primarily involved with the planning and initiation of movement, especially those movements requiring precise and rapid dexterous limb motion.
Spinocerebellum	Receives afferent information from somatosensory, visual, and vestibular systems and adjusts ongoing movements through influential corrections with brain stem and motor cortex.

Feedforward and Feedback Controls

Control over the dynamic restraints, independent of the motor control level, can occur through both feedforward and feedback. Feedforward controls are the anticipatory actions that occur once the beginning, as well as the effect, of an impending event or stimulus has been identified, whereas feedback controls are the actions that occur in direct response to sensory detection of effects from the arrival of the event or stimulus[6-8] (Table 2). Both feedforward and feedback controls play unique but inter-related roles in control over the dynamic restraints.

The traditional view has been that the main role played by articular afferents in FJS is direct reflexive activation of α-MNs, thereby providing feedback control over the dynamic restraints. Most of the direct support for this hypothesis is from studies using direct electrical and mechanical stimulation of the joint ligaments and/or capsule.[9-15] Unfortunately, claiming that direct α-MN reflexes are natural physiologic phenomena based on these methodologies is difficult for two reasons. First, findings

Table 2 Control Over Dynamic Restraints

Feedforward controls	Anticipatory action that occurs once the beginning and the effect of an impending event or stimulus has been identified
Feedback controls	Actions that occur in direct response to sensory detection of effects from the arrival of the event or stimulus

obtained through electrical stimulation may not apply to normal physiologic function. Second, the mechanical stimulation studies have been criticized because of the relatively high loading required to elicit α-MN responses.[16-18]

In addition, issues arise concerning the practicality of sole dependence on feedback controls to provide adequate dynamic restraint activation to enable FJS.[17-20] Inherent to any feedback control is latency, the period of time between the detection of the stimulus by the system and the completion of a corrective response. Maintaining FJS following joint perturbation, however, requires time between mechanoreceptor deformation and not only the arrival of an efferent neural signal to the muscle, as is often measured with electromyography, but also the production of internal forces sufficient to counter the destabilizing external forces. Further, to effectively maintain FJS, the duration of the α-MN response must be sufficient to absorb the necessary energy, thereby protecting the ligaments from injury.[20] Based on what spinal reflex tests such as the tendon tap suggest about articular α-MN reflexes, it is doubtful that they meet the requirements of magnitude and duration. Thus, it follows that for the dynamic restraints to be effective in maintaining FJS, other mechanisms governing activation seem to be necessary.

Many studies assert that articular afferents directly influence γ-MN activation, a concept that appears to be much less controversial than the α-MN activation hypothesis. Several studies using traction forces smaller than those associated with tissue damage and nociception have demonstrated potent effects on γ-MNs by articular afferents.[18,21-24] Cutaneous and muscle afferents also have been found to exert similar effects.[22]

The Role of Muscle Stiffness

Increased γ-MN activation has a multifaceted effect on FJS. Because γ-MNs innervate the peripheral regions of intrafusal muscle fibers containing contractile elements, their level of activation directly controls muscle spindle sensitivity and indirectly adjusts muscle stiffness. The ability of stiffer muscles to absorb additional energy from destabilizing forces may shield the ligaments from bearing the full responsibility of joint stability. Increased muscle stiffness, and, therefore, enhanced joint stiffness, is believed to augment FJS through an elevated potential to resist sudden joint displacements more effectively.[17,25-27] In joints that are mechanically unstable because of ligamentous laxity, stiffer muscles may assist in maintaining FJS, thereby reducing the incidence of joint subluxations.

Muscle stiffness, specifically defined as the ratio of change in force per change in length,[17,20,27,28] is largely dictated by sensitivity of the muscle spindles. Three types of factors contribute to muscle stiffness: passive, intrinsic, and extrinsic (reflexive).[29] The passive component is the viscoelastic contributions from the noncontractile elements; the intrinsic component is the number of actin-myosin crossbridges existing at a given time. Reflexes responding to elongation of the muscle-tendon unit comprise the extrinsic component. Thus, initial resistance to lengthening by a muscle is considered to be a function of the passive and intrinsic components until the arrival of an extrinsic response.

Increased γ-MN activation heightens muscle spindle sensitivity, which increases both the intrinsic and extrinsic components of muscle stiffness.[17,22] The levels of activation existing within a muscle at a given instant are a function of both the preceding reflexes and the excitability of the γ-MN pool from peripheral and descending supraspinal influences.[17] Increased dynamic γ-MN drive directly heightens the sensitivity of the primary muscle spindle afferents to changes in length.[29] Additionally, intrinsically stiffer muscles are thought to transmit loads more readily to the spindles.[30,31] Coupled with decreased electromechanical delay—the time interval between muscle activation and onset of segmental acceleration—the potential effectiveness of extrinsic stiffness is greatly enhanced in muscles with heightened intrinsic stiffness. Thus, increased γ-MN activation is not only a form of feedback control but also plays a feedforward role by increasing intrinsic muscle stiffness and extrinsic muscle stiffness potential prior to the arrival of a destabilizing event.

The Role of Mechanoreceptors

Experimental evidence suggests that mechanoreceptors also contribute to supraspinal control over the dynamic restraints. Freeman and Wyke[32] reported changes in supraspinal motor program control of voluntary movements in cats following surgical resection of the posterior and medial articular nerves. They also reported alterations in postural control adjustments initiated from visual and vestibular sources. Because Freeman and Wyke's procedure did not disrupt the mechanical stability of the joint, it is hypothesized that the alterations developed secondary to the loss of local inputs to the CNS concerning stresses on the knee joint capsule. Similarly, O'Connor and associates[33] recently reported that joint deafferentation combined with anterior cruciate ligament (ACL) transection resulted in more extensive cartilage lesions than did either manipulation in isolation.

Conclusion

In summary, proprioception appears to play an integral role in maintaining FJS. The processes through which control over the dynamic restraints emerges are extremely complex and are poorly understood. The topic that may have the most relevance to preventive strategies is that of supraspinal control over the dynamic restraints. Several studies of motor control have demonstrated the critical role proprioception plays in motor programs for goal-directed behavior. The concepts developed in these studies need to be further explored to determine the mechanisms contributing to the activation of the dynamic restraints during execution of a motor program. Intervening at supraspinal levels may be the key to providing increased dynamic stability.

Fast Facts

Fact: Functional joint stability (FJS) refers to the joint stability required for normal performance during functional activity.

Fact: Neuromuscular control refers to unconscious activation of dynamic restraints in response to sensory stimuli.

Fact: Spinocerebellar pathways leading to the cerebellum more than likely provide the organizational core of supraspinal control over the dynamic restraints.

Fact: Stiffer muscles may assist in maintaining FJS.

Fact: Muscle stiffness is the ratio of change in force per change in length.

Caution: Further studies are needed for a more complete understanding of the mechanisms contributing to the activation of dynamic restraints during execution of a motor program.

Begin: Begin incorporating proprioceptive drills into conditioning programs.

References

1. Matthews PB: Where does Sherrington's "muscular sense" originate? Muscles, joints, corollary discharges? *Annu-Rev Neurosci* 1982;5:189-218.

2. Lephart S, Riemann B, Fu F: Introduction to the sensorimotor system, in Lephart S, Fu F (eds): *Proprioception and Neuromuscular Control in Joint Stability.* Champaign, IL, Human Kinetics, 2000.

3. Sherrington CS (ed): *The Integrative Action of the Nervous System.* New York, NY, Scribner, 1906.

4. Sherrington CS, Denny-Brown D (eds): *Selected Writings of Sir Charles Sherrington: A Testimonial Presented by the Neurologists Forming the Guarantors of the Journal Brain.* London, England, Hamish Hamilton Medical Books, 1939.

5. Ghez C: The cerebellum, in Kandel ER, Schwartz JH, Jessell TM (eds): *Principles of Neural Science,* ed 3. New York, NY, Elsevier Science Publishing, 1991, pp 626-646.

6. Ghez C: The control of movement, in Kandel ER, Schwartz JH, Jessell TM (eds): *Principles of Neural Science,* ed 3. New York, NY, Elsevier Science Publishing, 1991, pp 533-547.

7. Johansson R, Magnusson M: Human postural dynamics. *Crit Rev Biomed Eng* 1991;18:413-437.

8. Leonard CT (ed): *The Neuroscience of Human Movement.* St Louis, MO, Mosby-Year Book, 1998.

9. Beard DJ, Kyberd PJ, Fergusson CM, Dodd CA: Proprioception after rupture of the anterior cruciate ligament: An objective indication of the need for surgery? *J Bone Joint Surg Br* 1993;75:311-315.

10. Ekholm J, Eklund G, Skoglund S: On the reflex effects from the knee joint of the cat. *Acta Physiol Scand* 1960;50:167-174.

11. Guanche C, Knatt T, Solomonow M, Lu Y, Baratta R: The synergistic action of the capsule and the shoulder muscles. *Am J Sports Med* 1995;23:301-306.

12. Kim AW, Rosen AM, Brander VA, Buchanan TS: Selective muscle activation following electrical stimulation of the collateral ligaments of the human knee joint. *Arch Phys Med Rehabil* 1995;76:750-757.

13. Knatt T, Guanche C, Solomonow M, Lu Y, Baratta R, Zhou BH: The glenohumeral-biceps reflex in the feline. *Clin Orthop* 1995;314:247-252.

14. Palmer I: On the injuries to the ligaments of the knee joint: A clinical study. *Acta Chir Scand* 1938;53(Suppl):5-282.

15. Solomonow M, Baratta R, Zhou BH, et al: The synergistic action of the anterior cruciate ligament and thigh muscles in maintaining joint stability. *Am J Sports Med* 1987;15:207-213.

16. Hogervorst T, Brand RA: Mechanoreceptors in joint function. *J Bone Joint Surg Am* 1998;80:1365-1378.

17. Johansson H, Sjolander P: Neurophysiology of joints, in Wright V, Radin EL (eds): *Mechanics of Human Joints: Physiology, Pathophysiology, and Treatment.* New York, NY, Marcel Dekker, 1993, pp 243-290.

18. Raunest J, Sager M, Burgener E: Proprioceptive mechanisms in the cruciate ligaments: An electromyographic study on reflex activity in the thigh muscles. *J Trauma* 1996;41:488-493.

19. Barrack R, Lund P, Skinner H: Knee joint proprioception revisited. *J Sport Rehabil* 1994;3:18-42.

20. Pope MH, Johnson RJ, Brown DW, Tighe C: The role of the musculature in injuries to the medial collateral ligament. *J Bone Joint Surg Am* 1979;61:398-402.

21. Johansson H, Sjolander P, Sojka P, et al: Reflex actions on the γ muscle spindle systems of muscles acting at the knee joint elicited by stretch of the posterior cruciate ligament. *Neuro-Orthop* 1989;8:9-21.

22. Johansson H, Sjolander P, Sojka P: A sensory role for the cruciate ligaments. *Clin Orthop* 1991;268:161-178.

23. Miyatsu M, Atsuta Y, Watakabe M: The physiology of mechanoreceptors in the anterior cruciate ligament: An experimental study in decerebrate-spinalised animals. *J Bone Joint Surg* Br 1993;75:653-657.

24. Sojka P, Johansson H, Sjolander P, Lorentzon R, Djupsjobacka M: Fusimotor neurones can be reflexively influenced by activity in receptor afferents from the posterior cruciate ligament. *Brain Res* 1989;483:177-183.

25. Grillner S: The role of muscle stiffness in meeting the changing postural and locomotor requirements for force development by the ankle extensors. *Acta Physiol Scand* 1972;86:92-108.

26. Louie JK, Mote CD Jr: Contribution of the musculature to rotatory laxity and torsional stiffness at the knee. *J Biomech* 1987;20:281-300.

27. McNair P, Wood G, Marshall R: Stiffness of the hamstring muscles and its relationship to function in anterior cruciate ligament deficient individuals. *Clin Biomech* 1992;7:131-137.

28. Nichols TR: The organization of heterogenic reflexes among muscles crossing the ankle joint in the decerebrate cat. *J Physiol* 1989;410:463-477.

29. Sinkjaer T, Toft E, Andreassen S, Hornemann BC: Muscle stiffness in human ankle dorsiflexors: Intrinsic and reflex components. *J Neurophysiol* 1988;60:1110-1121.

30. Fellows SJ, Thilmann AF: The role of joint biomechanics in determining stretch reflex latency at the normal human ankle. *Exp Brain Res* 1989;77:135-139.

31. Rack PM, Ross HF, Thilmann AF, Walters DK: Reflex responses at the human ankle: The importance of tendon compliance. *J Physiol* 1983;344:503-524.

32. Freeman MA, Wyke B: Articular contributions to limb muscle reflexes: The effects of partial neurectomy of the knee-joint on postural reflexes. *Br J Surg* 1966;53:61-68.

33. O'Connor BL, Visco DM, Brandt KD, Myers SL, Kalasinski LA: Neurogenic acceleration of osteoarthrosis: The effects of previous neurectomy of the articular nerves on the development of osteoarthrosis after transection of the anterior cruciate ligament in dogs. *J Bone Joint Surg Am* 1992;74:367-375.

Chapter 8

The Influence of the Neuromuscular System on Joint Stability

Laura J. Huston, MS
Edward M. Wojtys, MD

Introduction

It is well documented that a female athlete is more likely to sustain anterior cruciate ligament (ACL) injury than is a male athlete while engaged in the same activity. Research has suggested that subtle differences in neuromuscular control and function may be among the causative factors.[1-3] Recent studies have shown that teaching athletes balance training, as well as how to jump, land, and cut in specific ways, may decrease ACL injury rates.[4,5] This suggests that neuromuscular control play   very important role in knee joint stability and protection.

An understanding of how the active and passive restraint systems of the knee function is essential to a discussion of ACL injuries in women. Under physiologic conditions, stability of the knee is maintained by the neuromuscular system interacting with feedback from ligament structures, muscle activity, and joint-surface contact forces. The ACL provides approximately 86% of the static resistance to pure anterior tibial translation.[6] However, forces incurred at the joint during physical activity are often beyond the capacity of the passive ligamentous constraints, thus requiring the addition of active muscular forces to maintain joint equilibrium and stability.[7,8] When dynamic stability is inadequate or slow to develop, large forces are placed on the passive restraints of the knee, and failure can occur. It is imperative, therefore, that the central nervous system and the passive and active restraint systems interact optimally.

For years, it was assumed that the neuromuscular systems of men and women were similar. However, researchers are discovering that they may in fact be quite different. Sex-related differences in the neuromuscular system may play a predominant role in the high rate of noncontact ACL injuries seen among female athletes. The purpose of this chapter is to review the components of the neuromuscular system and their importance to knee stability, as well as highlight sex-related differences in the neuromuscular system as reported in the literature.

Muscle Physiology

Muscles provide strength and protection across the knee joint by distributing loads and absorbing shock. The stronger the muscles are, the more likely it is that the muscles will be able to protect the joint from a potentially deleterious force. However, factors that affect the ability of the muscle to produce maximum contractions include the mass (or cross-sectional area) of the muscle and the ability of the subject to fully activate the motor units (neuromuscular efficiency). Men generally have larger (based on cross-sectional area) and stronger muscles than women, although considerable overlap exists.[9-14] Several studies have reported that sex-related differences in muscle strength can be explained primarily by differences in mass (or cross-sectional area) and not by the quality of the tissue.[9,13,15,16] In addition, it has been reported that men demonstrate greater neuromuscular efficiency compared with women. In a unique study, Komi and Karlsson[17] studied muscle strength, fiber composition, and neuromuscular efficiency in sets of twins, each consisting of one boy and one girl. They found that boys demonstrated more efficient neuromotor output during muscle contraction and more pronounced contractile profiles compared with their twin sisters. However, the study did not consider the individual's previous level of physical activity, a factor shown to have a profound impact on neuromuscular efficiency.[18,19]

Muscle Reaction Time

Several studies have found that the speed at which muscle force is generated may be a more important determinant in providing joint stabilization and preventing injury than traditional muscle strength.[7,20-23] In other words, an athlete who possesses more than adequate muscle strength will still be likely to sustain a knee injury if the muscles are slow to react to a potentially injurious situation. Therefore, timely activation of the musculature in response to joint perturbations appears to be relevant to the ability of the system to prevent excessive joint deformation and ligament strain.

Muscle reaction time (MRT) is defined as the interval between the onset of a stimulus and the start of an action potential at the intended muscle. MRT is a valuable parameter in determining how well a joint detects a disturbance and how quickly muscles respond to a stimulus or perturbation.[24] Several studies[2,3,23] have reported no difference by sex in lower extremity MRT in young, healthy subjects. Winter and Brookes[3] used an acoustic signal delivered through headphones to compare the MRT of the soleus in a group of young, active men and women and found no differences by sex. Wojtys and We[2,23] utilized an anteriorly directed mechanical stimulus at the proximal tibia to investigate lower extremity MRT in a group of young, healthy men and women, and similarly found no differences by sex in either spinal or cortical MRT of the lower extremity musculature. Electromyographic studies suggest that muscle fatigue adversely affects MRT by increasing the latency of muscle firing and creating less efficient muscular processes.[25-27]

Muscle Recruitment Order and Muscle Activation Patterns

Some female athletes appear to use different muscle activation patterns compared with male athletes, which may affect their ability to stabilize the joint and therefore predisposes them to ACL injury. In 1996, we reported differences in muscle recruitment patterns between elite male and female athletes in response to anterior tibial translation.[2] Female athletes contracted the quadriceps first in response to anterior tibial translation (quadriceps dominant), whereas the male athletes, as well as male and female nonathlete controls, responded to anterior tibial translation by first contracting the hamstrings (hamstrings dominant).

Many studies have established the significant role of timely hamstring activation in improving knee stability.[7,8,28-38] These studies suggest that the hamstrings work synergistically with knee ligaments to assist in joint stability and reduce the magnitude of net anterior shear. In other words, if the quadriceps fire without the hamstrings, the tibia may subluxate anteriorly and significantly increase the load on the ACL.[36,39,40] Conversely, if the hamstrings fire without a quadriceps contraction, anterior tibial translation is decreased and loads on the ACL are significantly decreased.[36,39-41] Thus, an athlete with a quadriceps-dominant pattern may experience significantly more strain on the ACL than an individual who simultaneously contracts the quadriceps and hamstring muscles or one who contracts the hamstring muscles before the quadriceps muscles in response to anterior tibial translation.

Differences by sex in muscle coactivation patterns in young subjects have also been investigated. Baratta and associates[7] quantified the coactivation patterns of the knee flexor and extensor muscles of nonathletic individuals, recreational athletes, and highly trained athletes. The high-performance athletes with hypertrophied quadriceps demonstrated strong inhibitory effects on the coactivation of the hamstrings compared with a group of nonathletic, healthy subjects. Athletes who routinely exercised their hamstrings, however, had a coactivation response similar to that of the nonathletic subjects. The study concluded that the coactivation of the quadriceps and hamstrings was necessary to aid the dynamic component of joint stability, to equalize articular surface pressure distribution, and to regulate the mechanical impedance of the joint. Baratta and associates suggested that high-performance athletes with a muscular imbalance could reduce their risk of knee injuries by performing complementary resistive exercises of the hamstring muscles.

Muscle Stiffness

Athletes appear to achieve joint stabilization by relying on some form of preactivated muscle tension in anticipation of expected joint loads as well as utilizing previously experienced muscle activation patterns and pre-programmed muscle activity.[42-46] This combination allows athletes a quicker and more efficient response in stabilizing the knee joint against potentially damaging joint forces.

Muscle stiffness is regulated by muscle spindle afferents from agonist and antagonist muscles with excitatory and inhibitory activity.[47,48] For the neuromuscular system to be effective in preventing ligament strain, muscle tension must be developed in a timely fashion. As muscles that span the knee joint contract, they act to increase joint contact force and decrease tibial-femoral displacements, dissipate ground-reaction forces, and possibly decrease strain in the ACL and other passive structures.

Muscle stiffness across the knee has both intrinsic and extrinsic components.[49,50] The intrinsic component largely depends on the number of active actin-myosin cross-bridges in the muscles at a specified time. The extrinsic component depends on the excitation provided by the alpha and gamma motoneurons. It is important to note that intrinsic muscle stiffness is probably the knee's first line of protection. However, the protection provided by the extrinsic component is potentially greater, and it can be modified with training. For example, Markolf and associates[33] reported that isometric co-contractions of the hamstrings and quadriceps could increase varus-valgus knee stiffness in nonathletes two- to fourfold, and that well-conditioned athletes were capable of increasing knee joint stiffness by a factor of 10.

Several studies have found that men and women differ in their ability to produce adequate muscle stiffness.[51,52] In 1988, Bryant and Cooke[51] looked at the varus and valgus stiffness of 17 female and 24 male subjects. They found that the knees of the women rotated 66% more than the knees of the men and were 35% less stiff. Such and associates[52] tested the knee joints of 70 men and women and showed that knee joints of women exhibited significantly lower values of stiffness than did the knee joints of men.

Electromechanical Delay

Apparent differences by sex in the generation of muscle stiffness may also be associated with differences in electromechanical delay time (EMD) and musculotendinous elasticity properties. EMD is defined as the time lapse between the neural activation of the muscle and the actual force generation.[1,3] This delay can vary depending on factors such as the fiber type composition and firing rate dynamics of the muscle, the velocity of movement, the viscoelastic properties and length of the muscle and tendon tissues, the activity state, and the coactivity of other muscles.[53,54]

Several studies have reported a difference in EMD by sex.[1,3,17] Winter and Brookes[3] compared the delay in muscle force generation in young, healthy men and women and attributed the differences by sex to muscle elasticity. Similarly, Bell and Jacobs[1] compared the EMD in men and women during a maximal contraction of the elbow flexors after a visual stimulus. Results indicated that the EMDs of the men were significantly shorter than those of the women. In 1978, Komi and Karlsson[17] reported that women have a 100% longer rise time in force development of muscles of the lower extremity. These studies suggest that mechanical properties within the muscle may differ in men and women, with men able to generate muscle forces significantly more quickly.

Table 1 Examples of Neuromuscular Differences Between Men and Women

Characteristic	Differences Between Men and Women
Amount of muscle	Women have less absolute muscle mass than men
Contractile properties	Less efficient in women
Muscle reaction time (MRT)	No differences by sex in either spinal or cortical MRT in the quadriceps, hamstring, and gastrocnemius muscle groups
Muscle recruitment	Women tend to contract the quadriceps first in response to anterior tibial translation
Muscle stiffness	Men can voluntarily increase their knee stiffness significantly more than can women
Electromechanical delay	Significantly shorter in men than in women

Conclusions

Several neuromuscular differences in the lower extremity appear to exist between men and women (Table 1). First, women have less muscle mass and less efficient muscle contractile properties, which may explain why women produce lower absolute strength values in the lower extremity than do men. Second, during training, female athletes are more likely to become quadriceps dominant, which may lead to increased strain on the ACL. Third, the rate of muscle force development is significantly slower in women than in men. Last, men are able to produce greater muscle stiffness across the knee joint. Collectively, these neuromuscular differences may help explain the higher incidence of noncontact ACL injuries in women.

Fast Facts

Fact:	Physical training has a profound impact on the development of neuromuscular efficiency.
Fact:	Muscle reaction time (MRT) is the interval between the onset of a stimulus and the start of an action potential in the intended muscle.
Fact:	Several authors have reported no difference in MRT between elite-level male and female athletes.
Fact:	Some female athletes appear to use muscle activation patterns that are different from those used by athletic men. Female athletes contract the quadriceps first in response to anterior tibial translation. This quadriceps-dominant pattern may place more strain on the ACL.

Fast Facts *continued*

Fact: Muscle stiffness across the knee joint may represent an important component of knee joint stability and injury prevention.

Fact: Electromechanical delay is the time elapsed between neuroactivation of the muscle and the actual force generated.

Fact: Women have less muscle mass, less efficient muscle contractile properties, a significantly slower rate of muscle force development, greater tendency to become quadriceps dominant, and less knee joint stiffness.

Caution: Differences by sex in muscle size, composition, and strength, as well as other factors that influence muscle function, MRT, muscle recruitment order, and muscle activation patterns are not clearly understood at this time.

Begin: Additional research is needed to identify why women become quadriceps dominant with training and to develop ways of altering this potentially injurious pattern of activity.

References

1.   Bell DG, Jacobs I: Electro-mechanical response times and rate of force development in males and females. *Med Sci Sports Exerc* 1986;18:31-36.

2.   Huston LJ, Wojtys EM: Neuromuscular performance characteristics in elite female athletes. *Am J Sports Med* 1996;24:427-436.

3.   Winter EM, Brookes FB: Electromechanical response times and muscle elasticity in men and women. *Eur J Appl Physiol Occup Physiol* 1991;63:124-128.

4.   Caraffa A, Cerulli G, Projetti M, Aisa G, Rizzo A: Prevention of anterior cruciate ligament injuries in soccer. A prospective controlled study of proprioceptive training. *Knee Surg Sports Traumatol Arthrosc* 1996;4:19-21.

5.   Hewett TE, Lindenfeld TN, Riccobene JV, Noyes FR: The effect of neuromuscular training on the incidence of knee injury in female athletes: A prospective study. *Am J Sports Med* 1999;27:699-706.

6.   Butler DL, Noyes FR, Grood ES: Ligamentous restraints to anterior-posterior drawer in the human knee: A biomechanical study. *J Bone Joint Surg Am* 1980;62:259-270.

7.   Baratta R, Solomonow M, Zhou BH, Letson D, Chuinard R, D'Ambrosia R: Muscular coactivation: The role of the antagonist musculature in maintaining knee stability. *Am J Sports Med* 1988;16:113-122.

8. Solomonow M, Baratta R, Zhou BH, et al: The synergistic action of the anterior cruciate ligament and thigh muscles in maintaining joint stability. *Am J Sports Med* 1987;15:207-213.

9. Behm DG, Sale DG: Voluntary and evoked muscle contractile characteristics in active men and women. *Can J Appl Physiol* 1994;19:253-265.

10. Kanehisa H, Okuyama H, Ikegawa S, Fukunaga T: Sex difference in force generation capacity during repeated maximal knee extensions. *Eur J Appl Physiol* 1996;73:557-562.

11. Hakkinen K, Kraemer WJ, Newton RU: Muscle activation and force production during bilateral and unilateral concentric and isometric contractions of the knee extensors in men and women at different ages. *Electromyogr Clin Neurophysiol* 1997;37:131-142.

12. Maughan RJ, Watson JS, Weir J: Strength and cross-sectional area of human skeletal muscle. *J Physiol* 1983;338:37-49.

13. Miller AE, MacDougall JD, Tarnopolsky MA, Sale DG: Gender differences in strength and muscle fiber characteristics. *Eur J Appl Physiol Occup Physiol* 1993;66:254-262.

14. Sale DG, MacDougall JD, Alway SE, Sutton JR: Voluntary strength and muscle characteristics in untrained men and women and male bodybuilders. *J Appl Physiol* 1987;62:1786-1793.

15. Castro MJ, McCann DJ, Shaffrath JD, Adams WC: Peak torque per unit cross-sectional area differs between strength-trained and untrained young adults. *Med Sci Sports Exerc* 1995;27:397-403.

16. MacDougall JD, Sale DG, Alway SE, Sutton JR: Muscle fiber number in biceps brachii in bodybuilders and control subjects. *J Appl Physiol* 1984;57:1399-1403.

17. Komi PV, Karlsson J: Skeletal muscle fibre types, enzyme activities and physical performance in young males and females. *Acta Physiol Scand* 1978;103:210-218.

18. Hakkinen K, Komi PV: Changes in neuromuscular performance in voluntary and reflex contraction during strength training in man. *Int J Sports Med* 1983;4:282-288.

19. Zappala A: Influence of training and sex on the isolation and control of single motor units. *Am J Phys Med* 1970;49:348-361.

20. Barrack RL, Lund PH, Skinner HB: Knee joint proprioception revisited. *J Sport Rehabilitation* 1994;3:18-42.

21. Small C, Waters JT Jr, Voight M: Comparison of two methods for measuring hamstring reaction time using the Kin-Com isokinetic dynamometer. *J Orthop Sports Phys Ther* 1994;19:335-340.

22. Walla DJ, Albright JP, McAuley E, Martin RK, Eldridge V, El-Khoury G: Hamstring control and the unstable anterior cruciate ligament-deficient knee. *Am J Sports Med* 1985;13:34-39.

23. Wojtys EM, Huston LJ: Neuromuscular performance in normal and anterior cruciate ligament-deficient lower extremities. *Am J Sports Med* 1994;22:89-104.

24. LaLoda F, Ross A, Issel W: EMG Primer: *A Guide to Practical Electromyography and Electroneurography*. New York, NY, Springer-Verlag, 1974.

25. Hagbarth KE, Bongiovanni GL, Nordin M: Reduced servo-control of fatigued human finger extensor and flexor muscles. *J Physiol* 1995;3:865-872.

26. Rozzi SL, Lephart SM, Fu FH: Effects of muscular fatigue on knee joint laxity and neuromuscular characteristics of male and female athletes. *J Athletic Training* 1999;34:106-114.

27. Wojtys EM, Wylie BB, Huston LJ: The effects of muscle fatigue on neuromuscular function and anterior tibial translation in healthy knees. *Am J Sports Med* 1996;24:615-621.

28. Aune AK, Ekeland A, Nordsletten L: Effect of quadriceps or hamstring contraction on the anterior shear force to anterior cruciate ligament failure: An in vivo study in the rat. *Acta Orthop Scand* 1995;66:261-265.

29. Hagood S, Solomonow M, Baratta R, Zhou BH, D'Ambrosia R: The effect of joint velocity on the contribution of the antagonist musculature to knee stiffness and laxity. *Am J Sports Med* 1990;18:182-187.

30. Hirokawa S, Solomonow M, Luo Z, D'Ambrosia R: Muscular co-contraction and control of knee stability. *J Electromyogr Kinesiol* 1991;1:199-208.

31. Louie JK, Mote CD Jr: Contribution of the musculature to rotatory laxity and torsional stiffness at the knee. *J Biomech* 1987;20:281-300.

32. Markolf KL, Mensch JS, Amstutz HC: Stiffness and laxity of the knee—the contributions of the supporting structures: A quantitative in vitro study. *J Bone Joint Surg Am* 1976;58:583-594.

33. Markolf KL, Graff-Radford A, Amstutz HC: In vivo knee stability: A quantitative assessment using an instrumented clinical testing apparatus. *J Bone Joint Surg Am* 1978;60:664-674.

34. O'Connor JJ: Can muscle co-contraction protect knee ligaments after injury or repair? *J Bone Joint Surg Br* 1993;75:41-48.

35. Osternig LR, Hamill J, Lander JE, Robertson R: Co-activation of sprinter and distance runner muscles in isokinetic exercise. *Med Sci Sports Exerc* 1986;18:431-435.

36. Renström P, Arms SW, Stanwyck TS, Johnson RJ, Pope MH: Strain within the anterior cruciate ligament during hamstring and quadriceps activity. *Am J Sports Med* 1986;14:83-87.

37. Walla DJ, Albright JP, McAuley E, et al: Hamstring control and the unstable anterior cruciate ligament-deficient knee. *Am J Sports Med* 1985;13:34-39.

38. Yasuda K, Sasaki T: Exercise after anterior cruciate ligament reconstruction: The force exerted on the tibia by separate isometric contractions of the quadriceps or the hamstrings. *Clin Orthop* 1987;220:275-283.

39. Draganich LF, Vahey JW: An in vitro study of anterior cruciate ligament strain induced by quadriceps and hamstrings forces. *J Orthop Res* 1990;8:57-63.

40. Dürselen L, Claes L, Kiefer H: The influence of muscle forces and external loads on cruciate ligament strain. *Am J Sports Med* 1995;23:129-136.

41. More RC, Karras BT, Neiman R, Fritschy D, Woo SL, Daniel DM: Hamstrings: An anterior cruciate ligament protagonist. An in vitro study. *Am J Sports Med* 1993;21:231-237.

42. Dietz V, Noth J, Schmidtbleicher D: Interaction between pre-activity and stretch reflex in human triceps brachii during landing from forward falls. *J Physiol* 1981;311:113-125.

43. Dyhre-Poulsen P, Simonsen EB, Voigt M: Dynamic control of muscle stiffness and H reflex modulation during hopping and jumping in man. *J Physiol* 1991;437:287-304.

44. Greenwood R, Hopkins A: Landing from an unexpected fall and a voluntary step. *Brain* 1976;99:375-386.

45. Leksell L: The action potential and excitatory effects of the small ventral root fibres to skeletal muscle. *Acta Physiol Scand* 1945;10(S31):1-84.

46. Thompson HW, McKinley PA: Landing from a jump: the role of vision when landing from known and unknown heights. *Neuroreport* 1995;6:581-584.

47. Johansson H, Sjölander P, Sojka P: Activity in receptor afferents from the anterior cruciate ligament evokes reflex effects on fusimotor neurones. *Neurosci Res* 1990;8:54-59.

48. Sojka P, Sjölander P, Johansson H, Djupsjobacka M: Influence from stretch-sensitive receptors in the collateral ligaments of the knee joint on the gamma-muscle-spindle systems of flexor and extensor muscles. *Neurosci Res* 1991;11:55-62.

49. Hoffer JA, Andreassen S: Regulation of soleus muscle stiffness in premammillary cats: Intrinsic and reflex components. *J Neurophysiol* 1981;45:267-285.

50. Kearney RE, Stein RB, Parameswaran L: Identification of intrinsic and reflex contributions to human ankle stiffness dynamics. *IEEE Trans Biomed Eng* 1997;44:493-504.

51. Bryant JT, Cooke TD: Standardized biomechanical measurement for varus-valgus stiffness and rotation in normal knees. *J Orthop Res* 1988;6:863-870.

52. Such CH, Unsworth A, Wright V, Dowson D: Quantitative study of stiffness in the knee joint. *Ann Rheum Dis* 1975;34:286-291.

53. DeLuca CJ: The use of surface electromyography in biomechanics. *J Applied Biomechanics* 1997;13:135-163.

54. Soderberg GL, Cook TM: Electromyography in biomechanics. *Phys Ther* 1984;64:1813-1820.

Chapter 9

The Neuromuscular Contribution of the Hip and Trunk to ACL Injury

W. Benjamin Kibler, MD

What We Know

Noncontact anterior cruciate ligament (ACL) injuries occur when the joint moment developed at the knee overcomes the static and dynamic constraint system. Based on scant research, the consensus of experienced observers, and videotapes of actual injuries, it appears that the "point of no return" position that develops the excessive moment is a combination of minimal knee flexion, some degree of knee valgus, and internal rotation of the femur on the tibia (see chapter 5, on anatomic risk factors). This creates, allows, or exacerbates the quadriceps muscle's ability to exert a force that can disrupt the ACL.

The Complex Interrelationship Between Muscles and Joints

Most research investigating the mechanism of noncontact ACL injuries has been directed at the knee. However, the knee joint moment actually is determined by the motion and position of adjacent links in the kinetic chain that operates during running or jumping.1 Knee joint stiffness to pertubation results from activation of both local and distant muscles.1-3 Therefore, the focus should be on the entire kinetic chain, rather than just the knee.

The biarticular muscles (ie, rectus, hamstrings, and gastrocnemius) play major roles in stabilization, force transfer, and force generation.[2,4] They transfer force efficiently from one joint to another because they extend one joint while flexing another. Because their total length does not change much, these muscles do little work themselves, instead transferring the developed force to the joint. The monoarticular muscles of the hip can generate force, which then is passed distally for joint stabilization or joint movement. For example, extension activation by the gluteii provides 21% of the quadriceps force to extend the knee in jumping, and knee extension activity provides 25% of the plantar flexion activity through the gastrocnemius. The reverse is true in landing activities.[5] Gastrocnemius activity and gluteal function facilitate the force required to balance knee flexion. Maximum efficiency of this biarticular force-generation/load-sharing activity occurs when the hip is near extension, so that gluteus activation is maximal.

Differences Between Men and Women That May Affect ACL Injury Rates

Several differences between men and women in biomechanical motion, positions, and force have been noted. Compared with men, women land from a jump with a more upright position of the hip and knee, with increased trunk extension.[6] This may appear to reflect increased hip and trunk extensor strength, but it actually is caused by relative weakness.[9] In the female athlete, the iliopsoas provides eccentric control of the hip and trunk during landing from a jump. Because there is little gluteal activation and less hip and knee flexion, the leg does not accept loads optimally.

Women also experience higher loads (force per body weight) than men in certain directions when landing from a jump[7] or upon executing a cutting maneuver (WB Kibler, unpublished data, 2000). These increased loads are in the anteroposterior, varus/valgus, and vertical directions.

Physiologically, women show differences in hamstring activation in response to anteroposterior pertubation[8] and in landing from a jump,[6,7] with the hamstrings being activated later than in men. Women also show a shorter duration of gluteus medius and gastrocnemius activation when executing a cutting maneuver, mainly in the stance or load-absorbing phase[8] (WB Kibler, unpublished data, 2000).

What We Do Not Know

Role of the Hip and Trunk in ACL Injuries

As with all the possible factors in the etiology of ACL injuries, the importance of the role hip and trunk contributions play is not clear. They may be fundamental, creating a "train wreck waiting to happen," or they may be only contributory (the "final straw") when other factors (eg, fatigue, loss of concentration, hormonal influences) are operative.

Differences in Muscle Activation

We are not sure what causes the differences in muscle activation. Is there a genetic component? Are they caused by differences in training or athletic activity? How important is fatigue? Are there other triggers (eg, mental or hormonal) to muscle activation?

Even if these differences are important risk factors for ACL injuries, what are the best indicators of their presence? Neither pure muscle strength or muscle imbalance testing nor proprioceptive balance testing appears to be accurate. Perhaps a better indicator of possible problems would be a subjective or objective evaluation of normal or altered segment sequencing, such as a change in hop posture while running or jumping.

Structuring Conditioning Programs

What is the most effective conditioning program to optimize muscle activation? Isolated muscle activation does not appear to be beneficial. Some sort of patterned conditioning, using monoarticular muscle facilitation of biarticular muscle activation in sport- or activity-specific patterns, would probably be most productive (Figs. 1 through 4). Emphasis should be placed on achieving better "athleticism" and on visualization of motions and actions.

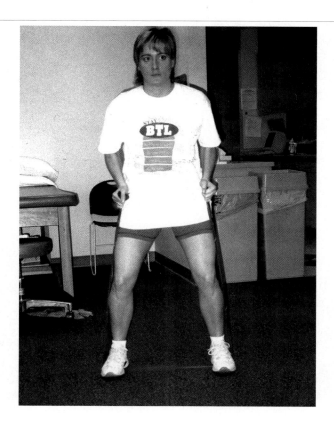

Fig. 1 *The joints of the leg are linked to create a balance between flexibility for load absorption and stiffness to give the entire leg stability. The athlete demonstrates load absorption on landing with minimal hip and knee flexion and by balancing the trunk over the legs and stiffening the entire leg to stabilize the individual joints.*

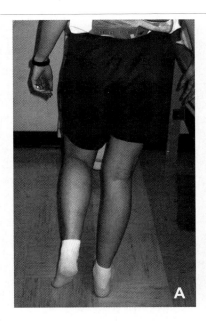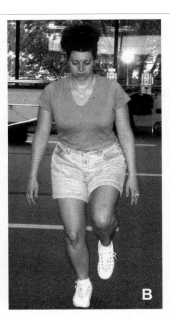

Fig. 2 The hip muscles assume primary importance by controlling the trunk in relation to the leg and by increasing quadriceps and hamstrings activation. *A*, The athlete shows the effect of weak hip abductors on the entire kinetic chain and leg: lateral trunk lean, dropped opposite hip, increased knee flexion, and slight knee valgus with internal rotation. This posture qualifies the athlete as "at risk." *B*, Strong hip abductors keep the body balanced over the trunk, keep the knee straight, and decrease the loads on the knee.

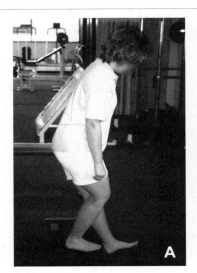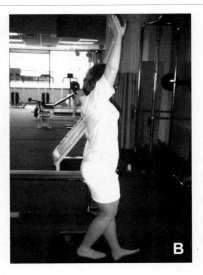

Fig. 3 A, The effect of weak hip extensors on the knee: increased hip flexion and knee flexion, with the quadriceps vector stressing the anterior cruciate ligament. *B*, Strong hip extensors decrease hip flexion and knee flexion, keeping the quadriceps vector within theoretically safe limits.

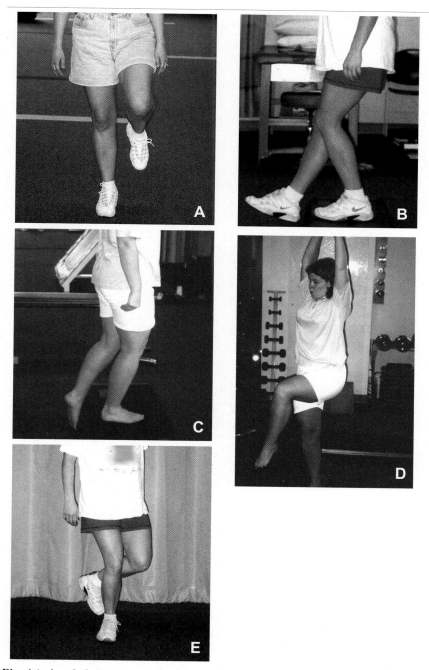

Fig. 4 *A closed-chain program should start from the ideal position of hip/trunk exten-sion, neutral hip varus/valgus, and slight knee flexion (**A**). All of the exercises concen-trate on maintaining this position while stressing specific muscles or joints up and down the chain. Among the exercises are step down (**B**) and step up (**C**) for trunk/hip control, and trunk rotation (**D** and **E**), which stabilizes against rotational loads and is an effective exercise to facilitate the vastus medialis oblique muscle.*

Fast Facts

Fact: Compared with men, women land from a jump in a more upright position, with increased trunk, hip, and knee extension.

Fact: As with other potential risk factors for ACL injuries, how major a role hip and trunk contributions play is not clear.

Caution: We are not certain what factors affect muscle activation, but genetic, psychologic, hormonal, and training factors have all been proposed.

Begin: When formulating ACL prevention strategies, consider conditioning all the muscles of the trunk and extremity, not just the muscles about the knee.

References

1. Putnam CA: Sequential motions of body segments in striking and throwing skills: Descriptions and explanations. *J Biomech* 1993;26(Suppl 1):125-135.

2. van Ingen Schenau GJ, Bobbert MF, Rozendal RH: The unique action of bi-articular muscles in complex movements. *J Anat* 1987;155:1-5.

3. Bobbert MF, van Zandwijk JP: Dynamics of force and muscle stimulation in human vertical jumping. *Med Sci Sports Exerc* 1999;31:303-310.

4. Gregoire L, Veeger HE, Huijing PA, van Ingen Schenau GJ: Role of mono- and biarticular muscles in explosive movements. *Int J Sports Med* 1984;5:301-305.

5. Umberger BR: Mechanics of the vertical jump and two-joint muscles: Implications for training. *J Strength Conditioning* 1998;70-74.

6. Devita P, Skelly WA: Effect of landing stiffness on joint kinetics and energetics in the lower extremity. *Med Sci Sports Exerc* 1992;24:108-115.

7. Hewett TE, Stroupe AL, Nance TA, Noyes FR: Plyometric training in female athletes: Decreased impact forces and increased hamstring torques. *Am J Sports Med* 1996;24:765-773.

8. Huston LJ, Wojtys EM: Neuromuscular performance characteristics in elite female athletes. *Am J Sports Med* 1996;24:427-436.

Chapter 10
Biomechanical Considerations

Donald T. Kirkendall, PhD
William E. Garrett, Jr, MD, PhD

Introduction

Many explanations have been suggested for why the incidence of anterior cruciate ligament (ACL) tears is higher in women than in men. An ACL injury can result either from contact to the knee or from some unexplained noncontact mechanism during sports activities athletes encounter every day. The fact that there are noncontact injuries suggests there must be intrinsic factors that can lead to ACL rupture. The mechanisms of ACL injury have been explored in depth in the sport of Alpine skiing, but little research has been done on other sports. In 1985, Feagin and Lambert[1] suggested that key elements of an ACL injury mechanism are movements that require sudden deceleration and an abrupt change of direction on a fixed foot. McNair and associates[2] agreed, based on their findings from their study of injury mechanisms in 23 athletes, and noted that 70% of ACL injuries were noncontact injuries, while the remaining 30% involved direct knee contact. Athletes who could describe the injury in detail estimated their knee flexion angle at the time of injury to be between full extension and 20°, accompanied by some tibial internal rotation.

Arendt and Dick[3] have determined possible ACL injury factors to be either intrinsic or extrinsic. They suggested that intrinsic factors included intercondylar notch size, size of the ACL, joint laxity, and lower extremity malalignment. Extrinsic factors included atypical quadriceps-hamstring interactions, altered neuromuscular control, possible hormonal influences, environment, playing surface, the interface between the shoe and the playing surface, and the playing style of the athlete.

The goal of the medical community dedicated to sports injuries is to prevent such injuries. Despite the significant attention that has been directed to ACL injuries, we are still at a loss to explain how noncontact injuries occur. Prevention of contact injuries is obvious: avoid knee contact. However, if we are to develop strategies to prevent noncontact injuries, we first need to understand how the injury occurs. Only then can tactics be developed to minimize exposure to potentially hazardous situations.

Injury Mechanisms

Duke Study: Questionnaire Analysis

Boden and associates[4] used a detailed questionnaire to determine common characteristics of ACL injuries. They analyzed responses from 65 men with 72 ACL injuries and 25 women with 28 ACL injuries. The average age when injured was 26 years; the range was from 14 to 48 years of age.

Contact was the mechanism of injury in only 29% of the patients; this is in agreement with other reports. The sports that represented the greatest number of ACL injuries were basketball (25%), football (21%), and soccer (21%). Injuries occurred in all levels of play: 41% during recreational play, 34% during varsity level participation, and 23% during intramural-level activity.

The overwhelming majority (nearly 75%) of the injured athletes heard a "pop" at the time of injury, and only three athletes were able to continue playing. The average knee flexion angle was approximately 20°, but the athletes reported a very wide range, from −10° to 110°. Removing the few hyperextension injuries changed the average knee flexion angle very little (to 24°). Movement at the time of injury included decelerating (34 injuries), landing from a jump (vertical deceleration; 30 injuries), accelerating (13 injuries), and falling backward (4 injuries). Nineteen athletes could not recall their movement at the time of injury.

The shoe/surface interface was cited as a factor in the injury by 21 athletes, 15 of whom said that their cleats were fixed to the ground. The remaining six reported that their shoes did not allow them to pivot.

While hamstring flexibility is thought to decrease the risk of strain injury, excessive hamstring flexibility might allow the tibia some additional room for an activity-induced anterior drawer maneuver. Boden and associates evaluated the relative flexibility of the athletes in their study. All but three players were able to touch the ground with their fingers, knuckles, or palms, suggesting that the group had good hamstring flexibility.

The interviews conducted by Boden and associates showed numerous mechanisms, which might fall under two broad classifications. In one classification were injuries due to tibial rotation, when the body twisted in a direction opposite the tibial rotation. The other classification included the 30 that were due to landing that forced the knee into an awkward position of either varus, valgus, or hyperextension.

Duke Study: Videotape Analysis

The next step by Boden and associates was to review videotapes of 28 National Collegiate Athletic Association Division I athletes and 22 recreational or high school athletes whose injury was captured on videotape. They compared their observations from these tapes to the information obtained from the questionnaire. There were no skiing injuries. Two out of three injuries were the result of noncontact mechanisms, though the athletes were usually very close to another player, most often an opponent, at the time of these noncontact injuries. While there was no direct contact with the knee in most of the injuries, there was some body contact that could have thrown the athlete off balance. Just prior to collapse, the foot appeared to be at or near foot strike, between 10° and 30° of knee flexion. Landing on one leg with that leg in valgus led to four of the noncontact injuries, while decelerating or pivoting caused the remaining injuries.

Role of the Extensor Mechanism

The work of Boden and associates[4] provides key insights into the situation surrounding noncontact ACL injuries and provides evidence that the quadriceps may supply the forces necessary to tear the ACL. The next step was to see if the quadriceps had the capacity to exert a sufficient anterior drawer maneuver to tear the ACL.

Patellar Tendon–Tibial Shaft Angle In 1984, Grood and associates[5] demonstrated that the ACL is loaded by the quadriceps through the full range of motion. Studies measuring the force on the ACL produced from the quadriceps muscles are usually done on cadavers in an open-chain setting[6-8] and typically show that the patellar tendon–tibial shaft angle is inversely proportional to knee flexion angle. However, for an accurate estimation of forces across the knee, the patellar tendon–tibial shaft angle in a closed-chain setting (when the foot is on the ground) is needed. Cadaveric data, though very well defined, might not generalize to the cutting or landing athlete. First, there is the difficulty in generalizing from the cadaver to the athlete because of internal and external validity concerns. Second, the patient interviews and videotapes suggest that these injuries do not occur in an open-chain setting. Therefore, an estimate of the in vivo forces on the ACL during closed-chain activities is lacking.

Noonan and associates (TJ Noonan, B Yu, WE Garrett, Jr, unpublished data, 2000) approached this problem by studying sagittal radiographs of the knees of nine healthy young men at knee flexion angles of 5°, 30°, 45°, and 60° (as defined by Winter[9]) while the subjects applied about 50% of their body weight. From these radiographs, Noonan and associates determined the vectors between the patellar tendon and tibia at each angle (Fig. 1), defined as the patellar tendon–tibial shaft angle. They found an inverse linear relationship between the knee flexion angle and the resultant force vector. That is, as the knee flexion angle decreased, the resultant force vector increased. Using published data,[6,7,10,11] Noonan and associates then used these measurements to estimate the shear force exerted on the tibia by the patellar tendon. During running and cutting, the resultant forces could exceed 2,000 N, which is very near the loads found in one study[12] to lead to ACL failure. When the quadriceps contract eccentrically, the resultant force on the patellar tendon at foot strike can be even greater, exceeding 5,000 N. These data are still limited because they were derived from men only and only for knee flexion angles between 15° and 60°. Research is needed to see if the same relationships hold for women, for a broader age range, and for a greater range of knee flexion angles.

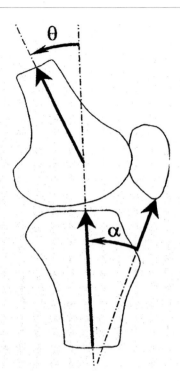

Fig. 1 *Patellar tendon–tibial shaft angle. The knee flexion angle, θ, is the angle formed by the intersection of the lines formed by the vertical axes of the femur and tibia. The patellar tendon–tibial shaft angle, α, is formed by the intersection of the vertical axis of the tibia and the patellar tendon.*

Kinematics The work of Noonan and associates showed that the quadriceps could generate the necessary force for an anterior drawer maneuver that potentially could exceed the force necessary for ACL rupture. A counter to this force must exist, or there would be even more ACL injuries than are presently sustained. The hamstrings probably need to be activated to protect the ACL from the high forces generated by the quadriceps. This suggests that there must be motor patterns that coordinate the firing of these two muscle groups to protect the ACL, especially during high-risk activities. There are likely to be differences between how men and women perform these activities, given that women injure the ACL more frequently than do men. To study these differences, controlled laboratory studies of men and women performing the same movements are needed. This would provide data to compare motion, muscle activation, and resultant shear forces during hazardous activities.

Malinzak and associates[13] examined differences by sex in the kinematics of running and cutting. They used three-dimensional motion capture to measure knee, hip, and ankle flexion angles and knee varus/valgus. Quadriceps and hamstring (medial and lateral) activity was determined using electromyography and reported as relative activation (the ratio of the activity of the quadriceps to the activity of the hamstring). It appears that women cut and land using a more erect posture than men. That means they have less knee and hip flexion and show more valgus at the knee (Fig. 2). The muscle mechanics of this position favors the quadriceps while denying a favorable position for the hamstrings to counteract the quadriceps. The women also had greater relative quadriceps activation than would be expected given the joint angles. Therefore, when cutting, women placed their knee in a position that favored a quadriceps-induced anterior drawer maneuver, placing the knee in a position of increased risk for ACL injury. More studies are needed to determine whether teaching women to play in a more crouched position would lead to fewer ACL injuries.

As previously mentioned, in many cases the interviews and videotapes indicated that another player was in close proximity at the time of injury. Could this mean that immediately prior to a cut or jump stop, a second player threw the player slightly off balance? Did this force the athlete to change the planned movement to an alternative movement? Could this change in movement pattern lead to a quadriceps-dominated activation when the hip and knee are in positions that place the ACL at risk? Much more research is needed to answer these questions.

Conclusions

Tearing the ACL requires either excessive rotation of the femur on the tibia or an anterior shear force. In the latter situation, quadriceps activation that is not counterbalanced by hamstring activation leads to the tibia moving anteriorly under the femur. The athlete usually describes the injury as happening while landing or stopping, or when planting to change directions. The knee is usually near full extension. Looking at other mechanics, as the angle of the patellar tendon and the tibial shaft increases (as the knee approaches full extension), the mechanical advantage of the quadriceps increases. The athlete at risk performs cutting maneuvers at or near knee extension (0° to 20°), with activated quadriceps not balanced by the hamstrings, with a knee at a flexion angle that does not offer a mechanical advantage.

Differences between men and women are seen: women perform these cutting and landing maneuvers in a more erect position (ie, the hips and knees are closer to full extension). Therefore, one might hypothesize that providing instruction to encourage the lowering of their center of gravity during cutting and landing, making it more difficult for the quadriceps to shift the tibia anteriorly, would reduce the frequency of ACL injuries in women.

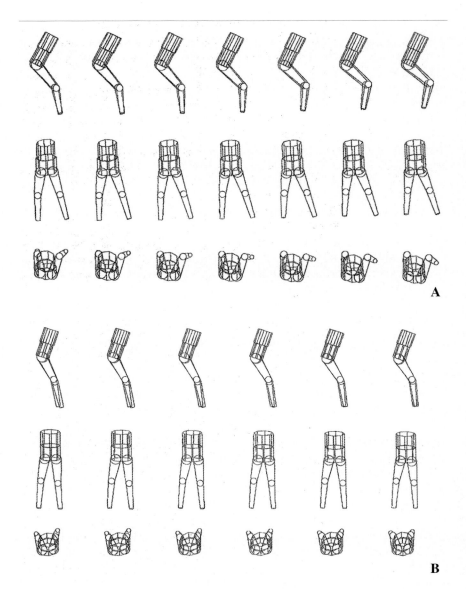

Fig. 2 *Three-dimensional kinematics of landing in men and women. Typical knee motion patterns of men (**A**) and women (**B**) while landing. The views represent sagittal (top row), frontal (middle row), and transverse (bottom row) planes. From left to right, the views show the horizontal movement component, from initial foot contact with the ground to the appearance of the peak proximal tibial anterior shear force. Women, on average, exhibit a peak proximal tibial anterior shear force 1.6 times that of men. Notice the difference in hip and knee angles between the men and women. (Courtesy of Bing Yu, MD, Department of Physical Therapy, University of North Carolina at Chapel Hill.)*

Fast Facts

Fact: Noncontact mechanisms account for 70% of ACL injuries.

Fact: Risk factors for ACL injury can be divided into intrinsic and extrinsic factors or into anatomic, environmental, hormonal, and biomechanical factors.

Fact: When cutting and landing, women tend to be more upright (less hip and knee flexion) than men.

Fact: Either excess rotation of the femur on the tibia or excess anterior tibial translation must occur to cause an ACL tear.

Caution: The role of perturbation in ACL injury is not clear. Further research is needed.

Begin: To decrease stress to the ACL, women should be instructed to lower their center of gravity when landing a jump or cutting.

Acknowledgment

This work was supported in part by a grant from Nike, Inc.

References

1. Feagin JA Jr, Lambert KL: Mechanism of injury and pathology of anterior cruciate ligament injuries. *Orthop Clin North Am* 1985;16:41-45.

2. McNair PJ, Marshall RN, Matheson JA: Important features associated with acute anterior cruciate ligament injury. *N Z Med J* 1990;103:537-539.

3. Arendt E, Dick R: Knee injury patterns among men and women in collegiate basketball and soccer: NCAA data and review of literature. *Am J Sports Med* 1995;23:694-701.

4. Boden BP, Dean GS, Feagin JA Jr, Garrett WE Jr: Mechanisms of anterior cruciate ligament injury. *Orthopedics* 2000;23:573-578.

5. Grood ES, Suntay WJ, Noyes FR, Butler DL: Biomechanics of the knee-extension exercise: Effect of cutting the anterior cruciate ligament. *J Bone Joint Surg Am* 1984;66:725-734.

6. Buff HU, Jones LC, Hungerford DS: Experimental determination of forces transmitted through the patello-femoral joint. *J Biomech* 1988;21:17-23.

7. Smidt GL: Biomechanical analysis of knee flexion and extension. *J Biomech* 1973;6:79-92.

8. van Eijden TM, de Boer W, Weijs WA: The orientation of the distal part of the quadriceps femoris muscle as a function of the knee flexion-extension angle. *J Biomech* 1985;18:803-809.

9. Winter DA (ed): *Biomechanics and Motor Control of Human Movement,* ed 2. New York, NY, John Wiley & Sons, 1990.

10. Huberti HH, Hayes WC, Stone JL, Shybut GT: Force ratios in the quadriceps tendon and ligamentum patellae. *J Orthop Res* 1984;2:49-54.

11. Perry J, Antonelli D, Ford W: Analysis of knee-joint forces during flexed-knee stance. *J Bone Joint Surg Am* 1975;57:961-967.

12. Woo S-L, Hollis JM, Adams DJ, Lyon RM, Takai S: Tensile properties of the human femur-anterior cruciate ligament-tibia complex: The effects of specimen age and orientation. *Am J Sports Med* 1991;19:217-225.

13. Malinzak RA, Colby SM, Kirkendall DT, Garrett WE Jr: Abstract: Electromyographic and 3-dimensional kinematic analysis of cutting maneuvers in men and women: Implications for anterior cruciate ligament injury. *66th Annual Meeting Proceedings.* Rosemont, IL, American Academy of Orthopaedic Surgeons, 1999, p 74.

Chapter 11

The Profile of the ACL-Injured Athlete: A Pilot Study

Elizabeth A. Arendt, MD
Julie Agel, MA, ATC
Randall W. Dick, MS, FACSM

History of the Study

Study Origin

In 1995 a representative from the National Collegiate Athletic Association (NCAA) Sports Science Division, along with a group of interested medical professionals including biomechanists, athletic trainers, and orthopaedists, met at the annual American Orthopaedic Society for Sports Medicine summer meeting in Orlando, Florida. The purpose of the meeting was to discuss various hypotheses regarding the etiology of noncontact anterior cruciate ligament (ACL) injuries in female athletes. The goal was to explore the possibility of a prospective study identifying variables that might be associated with noncontact ACL injuries. The physical examination variables discussed included femoral anteversion, foot pronation, knee valgus, and Q angle. Facts deemed relevant to the athlete's history included sport in which the noncontact ACL injury was sustained, years participating in the sport, day of the menstrual cycle at the time of injury, emotional stress or illness at the time of injury, and position played in the sport.

Regrouping and Pilot Program Design

The number of variables of interest was determined to be overwhelming. To reach statistical significance for even one variable, hundreds of athletes with noncontact ACL injuries would need to be enrolled. As noncontact ACL injuries are a relatively infrequent event in the college environment,[1] this kind of prospective study design would require taking physical examination measurements on thousands of athletes. The time and financial constraints of such a project would be prohibitive. Therefore, a pilot project focusing on a select group of these variables was conceived. The project was designed as a descriptive study, with its goal being "to determine if any of the injury, frequency, demographic variables, and factors were associated with occurrence."[2] In a descriptive study, data are collected only on injured athletes, not on the uninjured population. This research design cannot be used to determine association between risk factors and the occurrence of specific types of injuries because we do not know the rate of these risk factors in the uninjured athlete. In our study, data were collected only on those athletes who sustained a noncontact ACL injury, so only those anatomic features that could be assessed after the athlete was injured were evaluated. Our goal was to find any commonalities of abnormal physical examination or historical features among noncontact ACL-injured athletes as compared to general population norms, thus providing a profile, or snapshot, of the injured athlete. This would enable us to determine the most important factors to study in a more rigorously controlled, prospective fashion. In addition to attempting to identify common abnormal variables in the noncontact ACL-injured athlete, we also planned to compare features in male and female athletes to see if there were any differences by sex in these variables.

Data Collection

Interview

Two types of data collection forms were used for this project. The first was an interview-type questionnaire that reviewed medical and sports participation histories (Table 1). The athlete and the participating certified athletic trainer completed this form.

Physical Examination

The second form collected the physical examination features (Table 2). These measurements were taken from the contralateral limb. We felt that there was enough consistency in side-to-side measurement for the variables examined that measurements taken of the contralateral limb could be used as a proxy for the injured knee.

Directions on how to perform the physical examination features were given in both written and pictorial form. Phone consultation was available if necessary. The physical examination measurements were made by the certified athletic trainer.

Population Surveyed and Mechanisms of Surveillance

Data were collected from the 1996-1997, 1997-1998, and 1998-1999 academic years by certified athletic trainers at participating schools (Table 3). Initial communication site enrollment was accomplished through the NCAA injury surveillance system (NCAA ISS) network; also, conferences and colleges were contacted independently via the Internet. A telephone conference call that included one certified athletic trainer from each participating athletic conference was conducted in the fall of 1996.

Table 1 Questionnaire Variables

1. Mechanism of injury
2. Timing of injury: pre-season, during the season, post-season; during practice or game
3. Overall health of athlete, including mental and physical stress
4. Length of participation in the index sport
5. Bracing
6. Fit of athletic shoe
7. Sport and position played at time of injury
8. Diagnosis of injury and means of verification: arthroscope, magnetic resonance imaging, or physical examination
9. Prior injury to affected or opposite knee

Table 2 Elements of the Physical Examination*

Variable	How Evaluated
General limb laxity	Measured by hyperextension of the fifth finger beyond 90° at the metacarpophalangeal joint, hyperextension of the elbow beyond 10°, and apposition of the thumb to the volar forearm (ie, an abbreviated form of the Beighton scale).[3] If any of these variables was positive, the athlete received a grade of one. The athlete was considered hyperlax if all three of the upper extremity variables were positive.
Knee hyperextension	Calculated as heel height measurement in centimeters of distance from the table to the heel when the knee was passively extended. A measurement of 6 cm or less, which approximates 20° of hyperextension, was the value used to represent normal limits. It was felt that the heel height measurement in centimeters was an easier measure to reproduce than a goniometric measurement.
Foot-thigh angle	Defined as the angular difference between the axis of the thigh and the foot. This was measured with the patient in the prone position, hip at neutral position, knee flexed to 90°. This measurement has been popularized by Staheli and associates[4] to reflect the degree of tibial torsion. A measurement of 25° or less was the value used to represent normal limits.
Q angle, standing	Assessed as normal if 15° or less.
Hip internal rotation	Recorded in the supine position with the hip and knee flexed. This was used as a crude measure of femoral anteversion, as femoral anteversion is associated with excessive internal rotation of the femoral shaft. Internal rotation greater than 70° was felt to be significant.
Hip flexion contracture	Measured by positioning the patient supine with the lower leg dangling off the end of the exam table. The contralateral hip was flexed until the lower back of the patient touched the table. The angle between the long axis of the limb and the table was measured. Any measurement greater than zero was felt to be a positive hip flexion contracture.
Hamstring flexibility	Measured in the supine position. A measure of the popliteal angle was performed by attempting to extend the knee to 180° with the hip at 90°. A measurement of less than 160° was felt to reflect hamstring tightness.

*Performed on contralateral limb of the ACL-injured athlete.

Table 3 Results

Variable	Phase I: 1996-1998
Data sources	NCAA ISS; 20 NCAA and NAIA conferences cooperated
Population	97 athletes completed questionnaire
Sex	40 (41%) male 57 (59%) female
Diagnosis	19 by surgical verification 48 by MRI only 26 by physical examination only (orthopaedist) 4 by physical examination only (certified athletic trainer)
Prior injuries	Ipsilateral: 24 non-ACL injuries Contralateral: 30 injuries (10 ACLs)

Sport played at time of injury

Sport	Men	Women	Combined
Basketball	3	19	22.7
Cheerleading	0	1	1.0
Field hockey	0	4	4.1
Football	25	0	25.8
Gymnastics	0	3	3.1
Lacrosse	2	0	2.1
Soccer	8	19	27.8
Softball	0	1	1.0
Volleyball	0	10	10.3
Wrestling	2	0	2.1
Total	**40**	**57**	**100**

Timing of injury

	Pre-season	During season	Post-season	Total
Practice	21	18	2	4
Game	3	34	0	37
Total	**24**	**52**	**2**	**78**

Ankle bracing or taping	41 (48%) had no brace or tape 34 (40%) had both ankles taped or braced 1 (1%) had the ipsilateral ankle taped 3 (4%) had the contralateral ankle taped
Fit of shoe	5%: looser shoe fit 84%: average or tighter shoe fit 3%: very tight fit

NCAA ISS = National Collegiate Athletic Association Injury Surveillance System
NAIA = National Association of Intercollegiate Athletics
MRI = magnetic resonance imaging
ACL = anterior cruciate ligament

Phase II: 1998-1999

1,024 NCAA-sponsored schools contacted
371 responded
19 refused

118 noncontact ACL injuries identified
69 athletes completed questionnaires
45 provided limited or no data
4 refused

Responders: 9 (13%) male; 60 (87%) female
Limited responders: 6 (18%) male; 25 (76%) female

30 by surgical verification, with or without MRI
29 by MRI only
10 by physical examination only (orthopaedist)

Ipsilateral: 6 non-ACL injuries
Contralateral: 13 injuries (9 ACLs)

Basketball

	Pre-season	During season	Post-season	Total
Practice	10	33	1	44
Game	1	24	0	25
Total	**11**	**57**	**0**	**69**

44 (64%) had no brace or tape
18 (26%) had both ankles taped or braced
2 (3%) had the ipsilateral ankle taped
2 (3%) had the contralateral ankle taped

14%: looser shoe fit
85%: average or tighter shoe fit
1%: very tight fit

Table 3 Results *continued*

Variable	Phase I: 1996-1998
Health	77% had no injury or illness Body mass index not available
Mechanism of injury	Landing: 28 Planting/pivoting: 55 Decelerating: 8 Pushing off for jump: 3 Hyperextension: 10 Unsure: 3
History of participation in the index sport	
High school	93% played index sport for 4 y in high school 7% (2 men and 5 women) did not play in high school 6 men and 8 women played < 4 y in high school
Community	6.6 y (men) 6.71 y (women)
Age began sport	9.56 y (same for men and women)
Physical examination findings (contralateral limb)	68 athletes examined
Laxity	None had upper extremity laxity
Hamstring tightness	23 (33%) had tight hamstrings: 10 men, 13 women
Knee hyperextension	10 (15%) had knee hyperextension: 4 men, 6 women
Abnormal Q angle	8% (all women)
Tibial torsion	2 (2%): 1 man, 1 woman
Femoral anteversion	Results were unusable
Hip flexion angle	Mean: 177

NCAA ISS = National Collegiate Athletic Association Injury Surveillance System
NAIA = National Association of Intercollegiate Athletics
MRI = magnetic resonance imaging
ACL = anterior cruciate ligament

Phase II: 1998-1999

86% had no injury or illness
Body mass index 22.7 (18 to 36, SD 2.6)

Landing: 17
Planting/pivoting: 29
Decelerating: 17
Pushing off for jump: 7
Hyperextension: 7
Unsure: 4

98% played basketball for 4 y in high school
1 woman did not play high school basketball
2 women played < 4 y of high
   school basketball

62% played basketball in community
5.5 y

9.42 y: 8.22 y (male); 9.60 y (female)

66 athletes examined

12 (18%) had upper extremity laxity: 3 men, 9 women

16 (24%) had tight hamstrings: 2 men, 14 women

8 (12%) had knee hyperextension: 1 men, 7 women

Not measured

Not reported

Not reported

Not reported

Phase I

During phase I, which included the academic years 1996-1997 and 1997-1998, information was collected from athletes participating in a variety of sports. We decided that 97 of the injuries reported were eligible for further analysis.

Phase II

During phase II of the study, information was collected on only one sport. Basketball was chosen because the game is played similarly by both sexes. In phase II, we deleted several variables from the assessment because measurements were reported to be erratic (hip rotation), uniformly normal (Q angle), or difficult to measure (hip flexion angle). (Hip rotation, hip flexion, and foot-thigh progression angle were deleted because the measurements provided earlier were unreliable.)

Study Conclusions

The profile of the injured athlete as ascertained from phase I data is reported in Table 4. All conclusions reached in phase I held true for phase II, which dealt with only basketball. However, we could not draw a meaningful comparison between the sexes because so few noncontact ACL injuries were reported in men. Based on our data and the foregoing conclusions, we believe the physical examination features we examined are unlikely to be the variables that are predictive for noncontact ACL injuries in the collegiate athlete. Moreover, from this data analysis, we conclude that prospective measurement on a large scale of the physical examination features in our study would not help to determine variables predictive of noncontact ACL injuries.

Table 4 Profile of the Injured Athlete: Phase I Conclusions

- The most common mechanisms of noncontact ACL injury in the collegiate athlete were pivoting and landing from a jump.

- There was no evidence of co-morbidity of injury or illness at the time of a noncontact ACL injury in the collegiate athlete.

- The injured athletes were experienced in their index sports, with several years of participation prior to and during high school. There was no difference by sex in the experience level of injured athletes, as judged by either years of participation in their index sport or the age they began to play that sport.

- No consistent abnormal physical examination feature was found. In phase I, 33%, and in phase II, 24% of the athletes had some degree of hamstring tightness, as evidenced by a popliteal angle less than 160°.

- The noncontact ACL-injured collegiate athlete infrequently shows evidence of hyperlaxity syndrome.

Additionally, we believe that experience, as judged by exposure to the sport, is not a reason for the difference in incidence of noncontact ACL injuries between the sexes. Equivalent exposure to sport does not rule out differences in how boys and girls are trained. This may be an important factor we did not investigate. However, based on our data, lack of exposure to a sport at a young age does not account for the higher incidence of noncontact ACL injuries in women.

Fast Facts

Fact: The most common mechanisms of noncontact ACL injuries appear to be pivoting or landing a jump.

Fact: According to an NCAA study, laxity or other physical examination features such as knee valgus, foot pronation, or femoral anteversion do not seem to be predictive of a noncontact ACL injury in collegiate female athletes.

Fact: The number of years playing a sport does not appear to influence the likelihood of a player sustaining an ACL noncontact injury.

Caution: Prospective measurements on a large scale of physical examination features such as those surveyed in this study are unlikely to yield productive suggestions regarding avoiding ACL injury.

Begin: Institute programs to heighten athletes' awareness that pivoting and landing a jump are common mechanisms of ACL injury.

References

1. Arendt E, Dick R: Knee injury patterns among men and women in collegiate basketball and soccer: NCAA data and review of literature. *Am J Sports Med* 1995;23:694-701.

2. Schootman M, Powell JW, Torner JC: Study designs and potential biases in sports injury research: The case-control study. *Sports Med* 1994;19:22-37.

3. Beighton P, Solomon L, Soskolne CL: Articular mobility in an African population. *Ann Rheum Dis* 1973;32:413-418.

4. Staheli LT, Corbett M, Wyss C, King H: Lower-extremity rotational problems in children: Normal values to guide management. *J Bone Joint Surg Am* 1985;67:39-47.

Chapter 12
Video Analysis of ACL Injuries

Carol C. Teitz, MD

Introduction

To get a more accurate concept of the possible contribution of body position to noncontact anterior cruciate ligament (ACL) injury, a group of orthopaedic surgeons collected videos of athletes sustaining ACL injuries and did a multicenter analysis of these videos in 1998. We sorted individual film clips by sport, slowed them to the same speed, and included some "freeze frames" around the precise moment of injury. The group developed standardized recording forms that included questions pertaining to activity and body position at the time of injury (Fig. 1). We tallied the responses for consensus, defined as agreement by more than half of the respondents on what they saw. Questions were tallied as "no consensus" when there were multiple responses or when the observers were evenly split between two responses.

Results

Overview

The videotape included clips of 54 athletes, including 23 women, sustaining ACL injuries while participating in a variety of sports (Table 1). However, only basketball had a sufficient number of noncontact ACL injuries in both men and women to analyze.

Basketball Analysis

Six viewers reported on 22 video clips of ACL injuries sustained in basketball players. Because the mechanism of injury was not clear to two or more viewers or because the injury resulted from contact, eight of the clips were removed from analysis.

Data from the 14 remaining noncontact injuries are presented in Tables 2 through 5. Only three male basketball players are represented. Observers

Clip # _____
School _____

Sport	☐ basketball	☐ football	☐ soccer
	☐ volleyball	☐ other	
Sex	☐ male	☐ female	
Knee injured	☐ right	☐ left	

The following questions refer to the moment of injury.

At what time (as indicated on the tape) do you think the injury occurred?			
Contact	☐ yes	☐ no	☐ cannot tell
Non-contact but balance disruption	☐ yes	☐ no	
Off balance due to collision	☐ yes	☐ no	
Non-contact mechanism: stop	☐ two-footed jump stop	☐ Decelerating running without jump stop	
Non-contact mechanism: pivot	☐ toward injured leg	☐ away from injured leg	
Non-contact mechanism: landing from a jump	☐ no contact	☐ landing on someone's foot	

The following questions refer to the injured extremity at the moment of injury.

Center of gravity	☐ in front of knee	☐ over knee	☐ behind knee
	☐ to the side of injury	☐ away from side of injury	☐ cannot tell
Relative to trunk, thigh is	☐ adducted	☐ abducted	☐ flexed
	☐ extended	☐ cannot tell	
Relative to thigh, knee is in	☐ valgus	☐ varus	☐ no angular deformity
	☐ cannot tell		
Knee is in	☐ full extension	☐ 0°-30° flexion	☐ 30°-60° flexion
	☐ 60°-90° flexion	☐ >90° flexion	☐ cannot tell
Relative to the knee, foot is	☐ internally rotated	☐ externally rotated	☐ straight ahead
	☐ cannot tell		
Ground contact	☐ both feet	☐ only foot on injured side	☐ cannot tell
Ground contact on injured side	☐ foot flat	☐ on toes	☐ on heel

Comments or your narrative description of the injury

Name of viewer: _____

Fig. 1 *ACL video analysis recording form.*

Table 1 Sports and Number of Injured Athletes

Sport	Men	Women	Total Number of Injuries
Basketball	5	15	22 *
Football	18		18
Soccer	5	4	9
Volleyball		2	2
Gymnastics		1	1
Cheerleading		1	1
Lacrosse	1		1

*In two of the clips the observers could not agree on the sex of the athlete.

agreed that all the injuries in men involved landing a jump, whereas roughly half the women were injured landing a jump and half were injured when they stopped suddenly while running down the basketball court. Observers agreed that the center of gravity was behind the knee and both feet were in contact with the playing surface in 2 of the 3 men and 8 of the 11 women. Ground contact on the injured extremity was made with the foot flat in 8 of the injured female athletes and in all 3 of the injured male athletes.

Discussion

As exemplified by the lack of total consensus on the sex of the injured athletes, observer error must be considered in this analysis. Nevertheless, some patterns do emerge from the analysis of these videotapes. In basketball, recurring themes for mechanism of injury include landing a jump or stopping a run. Having the center of gravity behind the knee also was noted in two thirds of the injuries. Finally, ground contact on the entire foot ("foot-flat position") was noted in two thirds of the injured women and all of the injured men. The common knee position at the time of injury is knee flexion less than 30°, knee valgus, and external rotation of the foot relative to the knee.

Conclusions

The Center of Gravity: A Key Factor

The location of the athlete's center of gravity at the time of injury may be the key factor in noncontact ACL injuries. In the majority of basketball videos, the athlete's center of gravity was behind the knees at the moment of injury, not in front of the knees as one might expect given the forward momentum of an athlete running across a basketball floor. Similarly, one would expect an athlete to land a jump either bent forward or at least upright, rather than with the trunk behind the knee. If athletes made ground contact on their toes

Table 2 Mechanisms of Noncontact Injuries in 11 Female Basketball Players

	Number	Percent
Balance disruption	3	27
Off balance due to collision	0	0
Stopping	6	55
Landing a jump	6	55
Pivoting	0	0
Center of gravity behind knee	7	64

Table 3 Mechanisms of Noncontact Injuries in 3 Male Basketball Players

	Number	Percent
Balance disruption	1	33
Off balance due to collision	0	0
Stopping	1	33
Landing a jump	3	100
Pivoting	0	0
Center of gravity behind knee	2	67

Table 4 Position of the Lower Extremity in 11 Noncontact ACL Injuries in Female Basketball Players

	Number	Percent
Relative to trunk, thigh is flexed	7	64
Relative to thigh, knee is in valgus	8	73
Knee is in 0° to 30° of flexion	6	55
Relative to knee, foot is externally rotated	6	55
Ground contact with both feet	8	73
Ground contact on injured side with the foot flat	8	73

Table 5 Position of the Lower Extremity in Noncontact ACL Injuries in 3 Male Basketball Players

	Number	Percent
Relative to trunk, thigh is flexed	1	33
Relative to thigh, knee is in valgus	1	33
Knee is in 0° to 30° of flexion	2	67
Relative to knee, foot is externally rotated	1	33
Ground contact with both feet	2	67
Ground contact on injured side with the foot flat	3	100

rather than in a foot-flat position, it would be virtually impossible for the center of gravity to be behind the knee.

How might this errant center of gravity contribute to ACL tears? In the proposed "phantom foot mechanism" for ACL tears in Alpine skiers, the initial problem is that of the skier's hips falling below the knees, thereby moving the center of gravity backward.[1] The ski then acts as a lever arm to rotate the tibia and strain the ACL. In basketball, when the center of gravity falls behind the knee, the rectus femoris, acting as a hip flexor, may fire in an attempt to bring the trunk forward but overpull at its tibial insertion instead.

Prevention Strategies

To help keep the center of gravity in front of or over the knee, athletes should practice staying on the ball of the foot. Secondly, one should emphasize strengthening of abdominal muscles and hip flexors, particularly the iliopsoas muscle. Furthermore, Devita and Skelly[2] noted that 44% of the work of decelerating while landing a jump is done by ankle plantar flexors. Therefore, endurance exercises for these muscles should be encouraged.

Position of the Lower Extremity

With regard to the position of the knee in flexion and valgus and the foot in external rotation, it is not known whether this position increases the risk of ACL injuries or whether the lower extremity assumes this position after the ACL is torn. Nevertheless, the former possibility must be considered because ACLs are torn in this position in football contact injuries and in some skiing injuries. Women might have a greater propensity toward this position anatomically because of the width of their pelvises and a higher prevalence of femoral anteversion with compensatory external rotation of the tibia. Strengthening hip abductors and external rotators might enable better lower extremity rotational and angular control.

Summary

Although it is difficult for observers to reach consensus on what they see when independently viewing videotapes of injuries, some patterns regarding the mechanism of noncontact ACL injuries in basketball appear.

- Landing a jump or stopping a run with the center of gravity behind the knee was associated with two thirds of the injuries.
- Ground contact in the foot-flat position was noted in two thirds of the injured women and all the injured men.
- The lower extremity position frequently noted at the time of injury was knee flexion less than 30°, knee valgus, and external rotation of the foot relative to the knee.

A neuromuscular training program that would include keeping the center of gravity forward (incorporating strengthening of the abdominal and hip flexors, abductors, and external rotator muscles) and staying on the ball of the foot (incorporating gastrocnemius-soleus endurance training) might aid in the prevention of noncontact ACL injuries.

Fast Facts

Fact: In a review of injury videos, the knee position most frequently noted at the time of injury was knee flexion less than 30°, knee valgus, and external rotation of the foot relative to the knee.

Fact: In basketball, injury to the ACL commonly occurs when the center of gravity is behind the knee on landing a jump or stopping a run.

Caution: Avoid landing from a jump, stopping, or changing directions in a flat-foot position. When playing sports, stay on the ball of the foot.

Begin: Encourage participation in a neuromuscular training program that enhances keeping the center of gravity forward (ie, strengthening hip abductors and flexors as well as abdominal muscles).

References

1. Ettlinger CF, Johnson RJ, Shealy JE: A method to help reduce the risk of serious knee sprains incurred in alpine skiing. *Am J Sports Med* 1995;23:531-537.
2. Devita P, Skelly WA: Effect of landing stiffness on joint kinetics and energetics in the lower extremity. *Med Sci Sports Exerc* 1992;24:108-115.

Chapter 13
The Henning Program

Letha Y. Griffin, MD, PhD

The "Quad-Cruciate Interaction"

Just before his untimely death in 1991, Chuck Henning, an orthopaedist well known for his research in sports medicine, focused attention on what he called the "quad-cruciate interaction" and its role in noncontact anterior cruciate ligament (ACL) injuries. He believed that when the knee is straight during weight bearing, the ACL acts as the major restraint of forward movement of the tibia on the femur, providing an average of 86% of the total resistive force. With contraction of the quadriceps, the tibia moves forward, thus tightening and loading the ACL. When the knee is in full or nearly full extension, the forward displacement of the tibia on the femur produced by the quadriceps is large, thus stressing the ACL. If the quadriceps contracts when the knee is flexed to 60° or greater, the forward movement of the tibia on the femur is smaller, thus putting a smaller load on the ACL.

Henning's Prevention Program

After analyzing 564 ACL injuries recorded on videotape, Henning concluded that 75% of the injuries were from noncontact mechanisms. Of the 84 injuries that occurred in female basketball players, only 7% were caused by a direct hit on the knee. The most common mechanisms for the remaining injuries were planting and cutting (29%), straight-knee landing (28%), and a one-step stop with the knee extended (26%). The most common play situations in the noncontact group of injuries included shifting while on defense, jumping for a loose ball, dribbling to avoid a defender, going for a layup, jumping and landing for a rebound, and attempting a blocked shot. Using this information, Henning formulated his injury prevention program, in which he had athletes change the plant-and-cut maneuver to an accelerated rounded turn, the straight-knee landing to a bent-knee landing, and the one-step stop with the knees straight or hyperextended to a three-step stop with the knees bent (Table 1 and Figs. 1 through 3).

Henning believed that young athletes are the most receptive to technique modification, and he therefore encouraged teaching his techniques to children.

Table 1 Henning's Injury Prevention Techniques

Standard Maneuver	Recommended Maneuver
Plant-and-cut maneuver	Accelerated rounded turn
Straight-knee landing	Bent-knee landing
One-step stop with knees straight	Three-step stop with knees bent

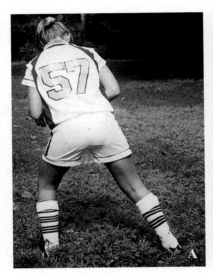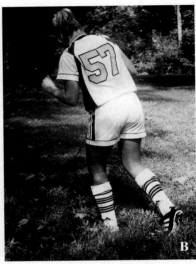

Fig. 1 Player demonstrating (**A**) the plant and cut and (**B**) an accelerated rounded turn.

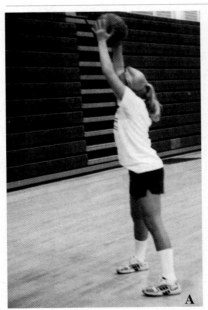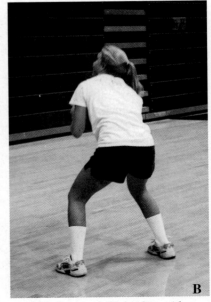

Fig. 2 Player demonstrating (**A**) landing with a straight knee and (**B**) landing with a flexed knee.

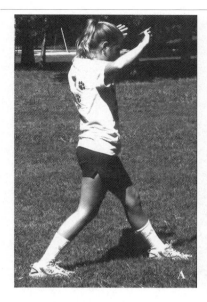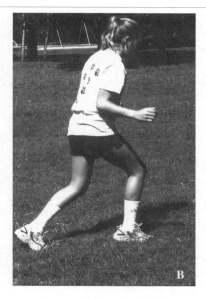

Fig. 3 *Player demonstrating (**A**) one-step stop with the knee extended and (**B**) three-step stop with the knees bent.*

Results of Pilot Study

Henning produced an instructional video that illustrates both practice drills in the gym and the application on the playing field of his three injury prevention techniques.[1] He instituted his program in two Division I basketball programs in the Wichita, Kansas, area. One team had incurred five ACL injuries during the prior two seasons (team A), and the other (team B) had incurred nine ACL injuries over the prior 3 years. After institution of his program aimed at improved player technique, the number of ACL injuries on team A decreased to two injuries in 8 years, or 0.25 injuries per year, and the ACL injury rate for team B decreased to one injury in 3 years, or 0.33 injuries per year, an 89% decrease in the rate of occurrence of ACL injuries.[2]

Conclusions

Because the study was not continued after Henning's death in 1991, the population tested was small. Nonetheless, these results are encouraging and are not inconsistent with the improved injury rates seen with the recent neuromuscular training program introduced by Hewett and associates.[3] Commonalities exist between these programs. Both programs teach the athlete to land with the hip flexed, the knee flexed, and the trunk balanced over the lower extremity.

Fast Facts

Fact: When the knee is straight during weight bearing, the ACL acts as the major restraint of forward movement of the tibia on the femur.

Fact: Henning believed that when the quadriceps contracts, the tibia moves forward, tightening and loading the ACL.

•When the knee is in full or near full extension, this forward displacement of the tibia on the femur is large.

•When the knee is flexed to 60° or greater, this displacement is less, placing a smaller load on the ACL.

Fact: Henning's prevention strategies stressed:

•changing the plant-and-cut to an accelerated rounded turn,

•landing with a bent knee rather than a straight knee,

•changing a one-step stop on a straight knee to stopping with a multiple-step stop with the knee bent.

Caution: Although Henning's principles seem logical, this program needs to be further tested on larger numbers of athletes.

Begin: Begin to incorporate Henning's prevention strategies into the preseason conditioning program.

Begin: Begin teaching these prevention strategies to young athletes to help them avoid developing techniques that put the ACL at risk.

References

1. Henning CE, Griffis ND: *Injury Prevention of the Anterior Cruciate Ligament* [videotape]. Mid-America Center for Sports Medicine, 1990.
2. Griffis ND, Vequist SW, Yearout KM, Henning CE, Lynch MA: Injury prevention of the anterior cruciate ligament, AOSSM Annual Meeting, Traverse City, Michigan, June 1989.
3. Hewett TE, Riccobene JV, Lindenfeld TN: A prospective study of the effect of neuromuscular training of the incidence of knee injury in female athletes, AOSSM Annual Meeting, Vancouver, British Columbia, July 1998.

Chapter 14

The Caraffa Program

Bert R. Mandelbaum, MD

Overview

In 1996, Caraffa and associates[1] published the results of their prospective study on the effect of proprioceptive training on noncontact anterior cruciate ligament (ACL) injury rates in soccer players. Their study was predicated on the concept that because proprioceptive training is essential to help prevent reinjury of athletes following injuries to knee or ankle ligaments, prophylactic proprioceptive training should decrease the rate of initial ligament injuries in these joints.

The Program

Caraffa's proprioceptive training program uses simple balancing techniques (Table 1). In phase I, the athlete practices balancing merely by standing on one leg and then the other. In phase II, the athlete does the same balancing drills but on a rectangular board. In phase III, a round board is used for the drills. In phase IV, the athlete alternates between the round and rectangular boards, and in phase V, the athlete uses a biomechanical ankle platform system (BAPS) multiplanar board (Fig. 1). Each phase also includes anterior and posterior step-ups. Athletes perform these balance exercises 20 minutes each day during the preseason (a minimum of 30 days prior to the beginning of the season) and continue the program 3 days a week during the regular season.

Table 1 The Five-Phase Balance Program

Phase	Type of Board Used for Balance Training
I	No board—balance on floor
II	Rectangular board
III	Round board
IV	Combined round and rectangular board
V	Multiplanar board

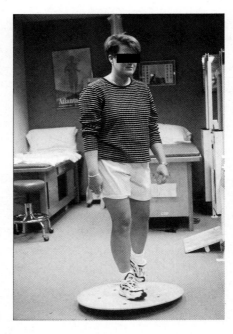

Fig. 1 *Athlete balancing on multiplanar board.*

Early Trials

To evaluate their program, Caraffa and associates added their balance training program to the standard training routine for 300 players representing 20 semiprofessional and amateur Italian soccer teams. Three hundred players, representing 20 teams, participated in their usual training programs.

According to the authors, the two groups were comparable in age and experience. The teams were followed for three seasons, during which time 80 arthroscopically verified injuries occurred: 10 in those who participated in the balance training program, for a rate of 0.15 injuries per team per season, and 70 in the players who did not participate in the balance proprioceptive program, for a rate of 1.15 injuries per team per season. This is a significant difference.

Criticisms of the study are that subject selection was not randomized and compliance as well as other program parameters were not standardized. Nonetheless, these early results are encouragingly supportive of this program, which intuitively seems beneficial. Further studies are needed to verify these preliminary results.

Fast Facts

Fact: Theory of Caraffa's program:

- Restoration of proprioceptive function is essential in ACL-injured and reconstructed knees.

- Restoration of proprioceptive function is essential following other ligament injuries, for example, ankle sprains.

- Exercises to enhance proprioceptive function should be included as a part of an ACL injury prevention program.

Fact: Caraffa's program was used by 300 soccer players in Italy, with 300 other players serving as control subjects:

- Athletes in the two groups surveyed were alike in age and experience.

- Results demonstrate a sevenfold greater injury rate in athletes not participating in the proprioceptive balance training program.

Caution: While institution of Caraffa's program at this time seems reasonable, additional studies are needed to verify the early results, as subject selection was not randomized and program standardization is difficult to assess.

Begin: Consider incorporation of proprioceptive drills such as balance board exercises into preseason and in-season conditioning programs for athletes.

Reference

1.   Caraffa A, Cerulli G, Projetti M, Aisa G, Rizzo A: Prevention of anterior cruciate ligament injuries in soccer: A prospective controlled study of proprioceptive training. *Knee Surg Sports Traumatol Arthrosc* 1996;4:19-21.

Chapter 15

The Cincinnati Sportsmetrics Training Program

Timothy E. Hewett, PhD
Jennifer V. Riccobene, BA
Thomas N. Lindenfeld, MD

An earlier study[1] has shown that marked neuromuscular imbalances exist in young female athletes prior to training. The study also showed that male athletes activate their knee flexors at three times the level of female athletes when landing from a jump, and it demonstrated that jump training corrects hamstrings/quadriceps imbalances, decreases impact forces, and increases strength and jump height. A 20% decrease in impact forces (or 80% of one's body weight) at landing is possible following training.

The Sportsmetrics Program

To prospectively evaluate the effect of neuromuscular training on serious knee injury rates in female athletes, we used a 6-week, three-component program (Table 1). The program frequency was three times per week, and it comprised a program with 20 to 25 minutes of careful stretching, a plyometrics training program lasting 30 minutes per session, and 30 minutes of progressive-resistance upper- and lower-extremity weight-training exercises. Weight training focused on closed-chain leg pressing.

Weeks 3 and 4 of the plyometrics program (the fundamentals phase) included vertical, forward and backward, and side-to-side low and high knee flexion angle jumps. Single-leg jumps that force the athlete to hold joint positions for up to 5 seconds were also incorporated into the program.

Jump training techniques taught included keeping an upright posture, with the body aligned with the chest over the knees over the balls of the feet. We instructed the athletes to jump straight up, with no forward-to-backward or side-to-side motion, and to perform soft (silent) landings using a toe-to-heel landing with an instant recoil for the next jump. We used verbal and visual cues with the athletes to promote proper form, such as "jump straight as an arrow"; "land as light as a feather"; "be a shock absorber"; and "recoil like a spring."

Twelve hundred sixty-three athletes representing 43 soccer, volleyball, and basketball teams from 12 high schools participated in the program and were monitored over their entire sports season. Three hundred sixty-six

Table 1 Sportsmetrics Training Program

Phase 1: Technique	Week 1	Week 2
1. Wall jumps	20	25
2. Tuck jumps*	20	25
3. Broad jumps, stick land	5 repetitions	10 repetitions
4. Squat jumps*	10	15
5. Double-leg cone jumps*	30/30	30/30 (side-to-side and back-to-front)
6. 180° jumps	20	25
7. Bounding in place	20	25
Phase 2: Fundamentals	**Week 3**	**Week 4**
1. Wall jumps	30	30
2. Tuck jumps*	30	30
3. Jump, jump, jump, vertical jump	5 repetitions	8 repetitions
4. Squat jumps*	20	20
5. Bounding for distance	1 run	2 runs
6. Double-leg cone jumps*	30/30	30/30 (side-to-side and back-to-front)
7. Scissor jump	30	30
8. Hop, hop, stick*	5 repetitions on each leg	5 repetitions on each leg
Phase 3: Performance	**Week 5**	**Week 6**
1. Wall jumps	30	30
2. Step, jump up, down, vertical	5 repetitions	10 repetitions
3. Mattress jumps	30/30	30/30 (side-to-side and back-to-front)
4. Single-leg jumps for distance*	5 repetitions on each leg	5 repetitions on each leg
5. Squat jumps*	25	25
6. Jump into bounding*	3 runs	4 runs
7. Single-leg hop, hop stick	5 repetitions on each leg	5 repetitions on each leg

Prior to jumping exercises
Stretching: 15 to 20 minutes; skipping: two laps; side shuffle: two laps
Note: Each jump exercise was followed by a 30-second rest period.
Post-training: Cool-down walk: 2 minutes; stretching: 5 minutes

*These jumps are performed on mats.
(Adapted with permission from Hewett TE, Stroupe AL, Nance TA, Noyes FR: Plyometric training in female athletes: Decreased impact forces increased hamstring torques. *Am J Sports Med* 1996;24:765-773.)

female athletes from 15 teams trained with the program; 463 female athletes from 15 teams did not train with the program and, therefore, were controls, as were 434 male athletes from 13 teams. All participants completed preseason questionnaires reporting prior injuries and years of participation. Certified athletic trainers tallied injuries weekly, completing reports documenting the number of injuries and injury risk exposures (one player participating in one practice or match). A serious knee injury was defined as a knee ligament sprain or rupture. All serious knee injuries were referred to a physician, and all suspected anterior cruciate ligament (ACL) injuries were confirmed arthroscopically. All medial collateral ligament (MCL) injuries were confirmed by physical evaluation, pain along the course of the MCL, and increased valgus rotation. No reinjuries were included in our statistical analysis.

Of those athletes participating in the study, 10 of the untrained female athletes, 2 of the trained female athletes, and 2 male athletes sustained serious knee injuries. The untrained group sustained five ACL and five MCL injuries. The trained group sustained one MCL and one ACL/MCL injury. The male group sustained one MCL and one ACL injury. These low injury numbers are the greatest limitation of this study, but it is difficult to generate greater statistical power with the relatively low knee injury rates of high school girls and boys.

The injury rate difference between female groups was significant at the 0.05 level using the χ^2 test. Untrained women also had significantly higher injury rates than the men, while the trained women were statistically similar to the men. The relative incidence per 1,000 player exposures was 0.43 in untrained female athletes, 0.12 in trained female athletes, and 0.09 in male athletes.

Serious noncontact knee injuries were suffered by eight untrained female athletes, no trained female athletes, and one male athlete. This difference was statistically significant at the 0.01 level. The relative incidence was 0.35 for the untrained female athletes, zero for the trained female athletes, and 0.05 for male athletes.

Noncontact ACL injuries were sustained by five untrained female athletes, no trained female athletes, and one male athlete. The difference between the female groups was again significant. The relative injury incidence was 0.26 in untrained female athletes, zero in trained female athletes, and 0.05 in male athletes.

Rectifying the Weakness of the Study

A weakness of this study is that the denominator (or the total number and type of athlete in each group) was slanted toward volleyball players in the trained group. Volleyball coaches have an affinity for a training program proven to increase jump height and improve net play and, therefore, they were eager to enroll their teams. No volleyball players in either the untrained or trained groups suffered serious knee injury. Therefore, we repeated the statistical analyses without the volleyball players to assess this study weakness. When overall serious knee injury rates were compared for soccer and basketball alone, a trend toward a decreased incidence in trained females was observed, but this difference was not significant. However, when only noncontact injuries were examined, there was a significant difference between the groups.

Conclusion

After the institution of the Sportsmetrics training program, the overall incidence of serious knee injuries in the group of high school athletes studied was between two and four times higher (depending on the inclusion of volleyball) in untrained female athletes than trained female athletes. Untrained female athletes were five to six times more likely than male athletes to suffer serious knee injury, but trained female athletes were only one to two times as likely as male athletes to suffer serious knee injury. These data suggest that a training program combining stretching, plyometrics, and weight training can be an effective prevention strategy for knee ligament injuries in the female athlete.

Fast Facts

Fact: Neuromuscular training programs can be used to alter strength and biomechanical patterning of the lower extremity.

Fact: Neuromuscular training programs have been shown to decrease the incidence of noncontact ACL injuries.

Caution: Although early results from the Cincinnati study on the benefits of plyometric jumping skills taught with an emphasis on proper technique indicate that such exercises are effective in decreasing noncontact ACL injury rates, confirming studies enrolling larger numbers of athletes are needed.

Begin: Incorporate neuromuscular training programs that include stretching, plyometric jumping drills, and weight training into pre- and in-season conditioning routines.

Begin: Include balance drills in sports training sessions.

Begin: When initiating plyometric jumping drills, emphasize proper technique: jump straight; land silently; and recoil like a spring, maintaining proper balance and body alignment at all times.

References

1. Hewett TE, Stroupe AL, Nance TA, Noyes FR: Plyometric training in female athletes: Decreased impact forces and increased hamstring torques. *Am J Sports Med* 1996;24:765-773.

2. Hewett TE, Lindenfeld TN, Riccobene JV, Noyes FR: The effect of neuromuscular training on the incidence of knee injury in female athletes: A prospective study. *Am J Sports Med* 1999;27:699-706.

3. Hewett TE: Neuromuscular and hormonal factors associated with knee injuries in female athletes: Strategies for intervention. *Sports Med* 2000;29:313-327.

Fast Facts

Fact: According to data from the Vermont Program, women have a greater risk of sustaining an ACL injury during Alpine skiing than men.

Fact: The risk of sustaining an ACL injury does not appear to be effectively reduced by improvement in the skier's ability or by increase in the skier's strength or experience.

Fact: Ski instructors and patrollers who formulated prevention strategies from viewing videotapes of ACL injury and near-injury situations sustained fewer ACL injuries than those in a control group.

Fact: Most ACL injuries in recreational skiing result from the "phantom foot mechanism." Elements of the phantom foot mechanism include:

- Skier off-balance to the rear
- Uphill arm back
- Hips below the knees
- Uphill ski unweighted
- Weight on the inside edge of the downhill ski tail
- Upper body generally facing downhill.

Begin: Become familiar with the elements of the phantom foot mechanism.

Begin: If the elements of the phantom foot mechanism begin to fall into place, one should keep arms forward, feet together, and hands over the skis in an attempt to avoid injury.

References

1. Stevenson H, Webster J, Johnson R, Beynnon B: Gender differences in knee injury epidemiology among competitive alpine ski racers. *Iowa Orthop J* 1998;18:64-66.

2. Ettlinger CF, Johnson RJ, Shealy JE: A method to help reduce the risk of serious knee sprains incurred in Alpine skiing. *Am J Sports Med* 1995;23:531-537.

3. *ACL Awareness— A guide to Knee-Friendly Skiing* (videotape). Underhill Center, VT: Vermont Safety Research.